BROADENING
My
HORIZONS

Living with Epilepsy

SECOND EDITION

P. J. Churchill

1

CONTENTS

3

Broadening my Horizons
Living with Epilepsy
SECOND EDITION

By: P. J. Churchill
Copyright © 2021 P. J. Churchill
ALL RIGHTS RESERVED
First Printing – July 2016
Second Printing - 2025
ISBN: 9781068975134

Acknowledgements

I would like to thank the following people who helped me compile and create this book. Being always grateful for their time and the information they provided me with as needed.

First, I would like to thank my parents for their unceasing help, and also to Dr. David Toorawa for his invaluable input and help in the collaboration of material for this book.

It is also important that I make a special mention of Professor Simon Shorvon, who played a major role in helping me put this book together as well as being my consultant. I would also like to thank Nick Kitchen.

If you like this book, please leave a positive review on Amazon. I would appreciate it a lot, Thank you!

P. J. Churchill

The Beginning

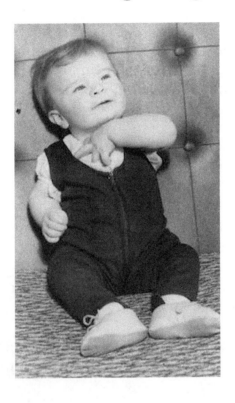

I was born in 1968 on a warm day at St Paul's Hospital, Hemel Hempstead in the UK.

As with all new parent's, they were overjoyed that they had a normal healthy baby.

No one suspected there was anything wrong until one day, when the convulsions began.

When I was about eighteen months old, and during a throat infection, which had been plaguing me; it was by sheer accident that I fell over and hit my head, then subsequently a seizure followed.

This convulsion was serious enough for my parents to need to rush me to Hemel Hempstead General Hospital. However, when my parent's arrived, they were told by hospital staff that there were no beds available.

The next closest hospital to Hemel Hempstead was Watford General Hospital. This meant my parent's had to drive an extra seven miles to get some medical treatment for me. All the while, blood was shooting up into my brain.

Tragic to think, that the time it took to drive from one hospital to the next had more than likely contributed to the beginning of my epilepsy.

From 1973, the Doctors had concrete documentation when I was admitted with severe epilepsy. Prior to that, I had Febrile Convulsions as of the age of 18 months old and again in early 1970, with no treatment.

In addition to that, I had absence attacks, however this was not reported until my admission to hospital in 1973.

In March of 1973, I was given a new medication called 'Phenytoin', when discharged from the hospital that year and this medication was taken for only six months.

My attacks were then also classified as 'Grand Mal Convulsions'. After medication, it was classified as 'Partial Complex Epilepsy'. That same year I was put onto Tegretol.

(I continue to take Tegretal to this date of this book being published.)

This was the beginning of many pills that I would be prescribed by my doctor.

School Days

Nursery school (kindergarten) that I attended was not too bad.

My first proper school was one called The Collett School. What I do remember is that whenever I had a seizure during my first year there, other children would tease me. They acted nastily because of my disability, hurtfully re-enacting my seizures by deliberately mimicking the actions of my body movements whenever they saw me.

The Collett School was a good school, but the many epileptic fits I had, did not help my education. Thankfully there was one upside to it that I liked being in the school plays, such as the Christmas Nativity play. Also at the time, as I was a fan of a well-known glam rock singer in the mid nineteen seventies, and an outfit was made for me to sing in the main hall of the school.

Unfortunately, on the day of the performance, I had to stay at home off sick after having seizures. I was so disappointed because in the end I never had the opportunity to perform in front of the audience.

That is when it hit home to me, that living with epilepsy, a disability was in fact interrupting plans at any given moment.

Making long term friends was hard, since I had taken to living in my shell, but I did have some friends that I would play soccer with whenever the epilepsy allowed. This was something I really enjoyed, but if my body got too hot through running about, then a seizure would be triggered.

This occurred about half of the time that I found at a young age, I was kind of restricted from running around the playground with my friends and enjoying all the activities when young children played together.

My ability to read, write and think plus make wise decisions for a ten-and-a-half-year-old wasn't a problem. When it was decided, I was to be transferred to another school. I had reached class five of the ten classes that were at The Collett School.

My medical condition prevented me from attending a school in my town, as at the time, no other schools in the town would take a child on with epilepsy, so my mother told me. Plus, my behaviour at home was not good either, due to the epilepsy and my mother did not fully understand everything about epilepsy at that time, so she decided to send me off to a boarding school.

It could not be helped that my epilepsy, was playing a part of causing me to be the naughty boy at home.

Every now and then, mother would ask relatives, like my nan or an auntie to look after me for the day or at times even stay overnight. This would allow my mother freer time for herself.

In January of 1979, I was sent to a boarding school in Torquay called Pitt House School.

Being brought up was not how it should have been by not being with my brother and sister at home and sent to a boarding school instead.

As for my health while at Pitt House School, things didn't always go well because of the epilepsy. For example, on one occasion while I was walking from the main part of the school to the playground area, which involved climbing concrete steps, I tripped and fell head first onto the concrete, hitting the corner of a step and cutting my forehead open.

Each term was about twelve weeks long. After a term was finished, pupils went home to their parents for a school holiday. It involved getting up at around 4 am. and getting washed and ready for the day of travelling.

We would dress into our 'flashy suits' that we would be wearing to go home. Had breakfast then collect our things and went to the front of the school, where coaches would be waiting to take us to Newton Abbot Train station.

The Pupils lived all over England as far north as places like Newcastle and Middlesbrough. I along with some other pupils from the school got on the train that went from Newton Abbot to Paddington Station in London. Some would get off along the way at places like Reading making the rest of their trip home by car.

Sometimes, I was met by my dad at Paddington Station, and I was always glad to see him. Then we would make our way home to enjoy the school holiday.

There was one particular school holiday that something happened, the exact reason 'why' or 'what' I cannot recall, but I did not want to return to school when it was time. The silly thing is that whenever I got back to the school, I settled in nicely with no problems at all.

There was one time that I did not return to the school until near the end of a school term, as there was only four weeks left out of the twelve-week term to go. I knew that I really did not want to return.

I had been away from school for so long that term, and I was going to be that unpopular with some of the staff. I found the prospect of going back even harder.

Things at school weren't always that bad and never really stopped me from doing the things that I wanted to do or liked doing.

I remember going ice skating when my parents came down to visit me in 1980. It was my very first and only time that I put on ice skates. I tried to stay on my feet while going around the ice rink, but was slipping all over the place, so just held on to the side as I made my way around the rink.

Since I also enjoyed singing, I joined the school choir and was at times chosen to sing a solo of some verses of hymns, during a Christmas concert. Those are good memories.

In 1980, I also had the opportunity to play a small part in the school play 'Tom Sawyer' being one of the boys playing in the playground.

In 1982, I was offered the part to play one of the main roles in the play 'The Wizard of Oz', playing the part of the cuddly lion. I had a lot of fun playing this part. However, on one occasion when I was about to go on stage to do one of the scenes when somebody deliberately stepped onto my lion's tail, and it came off the costume and had to go on stage without the lion's tail. To this day, I still do not know who did it?

Despite my efforts to take part in school activities, the epilepsy was still taking centre stage in my life. Plagued by these seizures, on many occasions, it prevented me from enjoying such things, like soccer.

On one occasion, we were having a good game of soccer, playing for the school team against another school team. I was passed the ball by another player and ran into the penalty area towards the goal with it and shot the ball passed the goalkeeper scoring for Pitt House School. I was in my elements and happy, celebrating my goal.

Watching the game from the sidelines was a House master and another pupil. The House master was heard to say to the pupil; "You watch, Peter is going to have a seizure."

Would you believe it? I did. I had a seizure, right there and then - game over for me as I had to be taken off the field and replaced by another player.

Another experience that I remember that involved sports was during a sports day not being a thin person you see. A few days before the sports day was due to happen, I asked the sports master Mr. McDermott, if he would put me into the 100 or 200 metres races.

When the schedule came out, of who was going to be taking part in what events, I found out that I had been put into the 800 metres race not the 100 or 200 that I had asked to be in.

The day of the sports events came and it was a lovely sunny day. Events taking place of the 100 and 200 metres races, High Jump and Long Jump along with others. When the time came for the 800 metres race to start. I got myself ready at the starting line along with all the other runners.

A teacher was at the start and shouted "On Your Marks, Get Set, Go."

So off we went, I started not badly, but was near the back after 200 metres. Found that I was getting out of breath and fell to the back and was now in last place.

The leader was well ahead at this point and the person in front of me was getting further and further away as I huffed and puffed. People watching the race, were cheering me on despite the fact that I was last and struggling.

I was not going to give in, so I carried on the best I could, reaching the 600 metres mark and everyone else being streaks ahead of me. Now I was running alone, running my own race. The leader rounded the final bend and into the home straight when I still had 150 metres to go.

Plodding along and gave it all that I could, eventually came round the final bend in last place and one final push to the finish line despite feeling tired and exhausted, making it to the finish line.

My legs were aching and I fell to the ground in a heap. I felt good and very proud of having stuck with it and completing the 800 metres, all the time knowing that I was going to find it very difficult to run, yet never giving up.

'Trip to Paris'

In 1982, I was in a house group called 'Star Group' along with the other pupils that were in this group. On one occasion, we went on a four-day trip to France, which included visiting Paris.

Driving along the motorways in France, as in any trip we had to make a rest stop, to me it was shocking to see that the toilets there were just a hole in the ground to do one's business through.

As we walked along the streets of Paris, smelling the aroma of roasted chestnuts that were for sale, I could not resist the urge to purchase a bag and share them with some of my classmates.

The highlight of our visit for me was going up the 'Eiffel Tower'. We went as high as the second floor from the top, as the top level was being refurbished. This did not stop the fantastic view from all four sides. The moment was very exciting for me, yet I was sad, as I did not own a camera and missed that golden opportunity to capture the view of Paris from this height and the street scenes. However, I am lucky enough to have a memory of this trip and views in my mind.

The unfortunate part is that I did have some seizures while on this beautiful trip. Yet, I did not allow it to ruin this wonderful trip for me.

~ ~ ~ ~ ~

In 1983, on another occasion during a weekend in June, when my friends and I were going to play soccer, I saw a well-known comedian called 'Larry Grayson'. He lived not far from the school and we would regularly see him walk his dog. I stopped to say hello to him and told him that it was going to be my birthday on the Wednesday coming up. He said to me in reply that when Wednesday comes, come to the entrance of the apartment building that I live in and wait for me. I said OK.

When Wednesday evening came, I walked to the apartments and pressed the buzzer and waited a little while for Larry to come out the door and he handed me an envelope. Saying thank you to him, I walked back to the school and went to my house master, Mr. Narramore. We opened the envelope together and inside it he placed a photo of Larry Grayson with a message written on the back of the photo which read; To Peter, Happy Birthday from Larry. He also had placed two one-pound notes inside. How nice of him to do that. I still have the photo to this day.

During my final year at Pitt House School, I gained work experience, as we had a teacher called Mr. Brandwood, who let pupils in their final year at school gain some work experience. By working at different places. I had a work experience, of keeping the grounds tidy at Torbay Hospital.

After doing that, I also did some work at maintaining the grounds and keeping area's tidy at Babbacombe Model Village. Another pupil and I also gained some experience in cleaning out dog kennels.

When the Easter term was over in 1984, I finished my schooling at Pitt House School. Was due to finish my school days at the end of the summer term and have schooling at home instead, which did not materialize.

However, my five years of boarding school were very interesting and taught me a lot in many ways.

Coping with Epilepsy
(The early years)

Childhood days were difficult enough, yet with the epilepsy *(depending what type you have)* you live with constant knocks and bangs. Cuts and bruises are always there to remind you of your medical condition.

There was an incident at home when I fell whilst having a seizure, right through the glass window of my parent's front door. I cut my head deep enough and needed to be taken to hospital and yes, stitches were required.

Like many young lads, I use to go to work with my father. One job he had was driving a dump truck. He also drove a tractor and spreader as he did chalk spreading for a company.

On one occasion while my dad was spreading chalk in a field on a farm, I had a close shave with death, as I rode on the back of the tractor.

Once the chalk was loaded into the spreader, my dad got out of the dump truck and climbed into the driver's seat of the tractor, and I was standing behind him on the back of the tractor. During one time that he was spreading the chalk around a field, I fell off the tractor, due to the fact that I had started to have a seizure with no warning.

Fortunately for me, my dad saw me fall and stopped the tractor immediately.

Otherwise, God only knows what would have happened to me if I had gone under the spreader and may have come out like mincemeat.

Every now and then though, when I was with him, he would sometimes let me actually drive the tractor and spread the chalk around the fields with dad by my side to watch over me.

For me to be doing this on these special occasions was very exciting and I was able to do so now and then for as long as dad had this particular job.

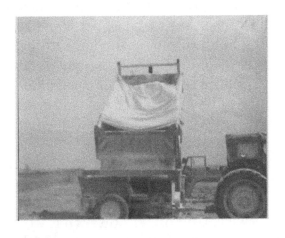

This is the chalk being loaded into the spreader before being spreaded onto the farmer's field.

There was another occasion when my dad was working for a salvage yard picking up cars from apartments and properties in different places.

While out on a journey to pick up three cars at three separate locations, he had one car left to pick up, when dad asked me to climb up onto the second car and guide him with the third car to place it on top of the second car.

It was then when a seizure started without a warning. I fell from high up and banged my shoulder as I was falling down the side of the truck and then smacked my head onto the curb.

I was out cold and unconscious, cutting my head open and blood gushing everywhere, in a way that head wounds would do.

In a panic, my dad rushed to the nearest apartment and asked those living there to ring for an ambulance and get me to hospital as soon as they can.

Within ten minutes the ambulance arrived and put me onto a stretcher and carried me into the ambulance.

They rushed me to the hospital, while everyone was very worried due to the fact that I was still unconscious.

Not long after the ambulance arrived at the hospital with me in, I came around. I had a dislocated shoulder and I needed stitches in my head.

My mother was not happy with my dad and from then onwards, he never took me with him again to work.

I can recall another day and another load of seizures that hit me. Of all days, it was my cousin's wedding day. To get there we had to travel from the county of Hertfordshire to get to Norfolk. However, things went wrong right from the start of the day.

While still at home and getting ready, I had two seizures. But it was during the wedding service itself that I had a seizure, causing the service to be interrupted. The wedding had to be stopped while they took me outside to get some fresh air and made sure that I was all right before they could continue the service.

"How embarrassing those moments are when it happens on a very important occasion."

Evening came around, and during the party I had more seizures, possibly caused by the flashing lights that were being used as part of the entertainment equipment.

Seizures may also have been caused by getting overheated while dancing the night away. Eventually and unfortunately, I went to bed early due to feeling tired and having three seizures in that one evening alone.

What a day! Overall, I had six major seizures in just one day. What a way to spend a joyful day for someone else's celebration and love towards each other on their wedding day. For sure that is something that will not be forgotten.

A Soccer Incident 1986

March 17th 1986 - It was an evening soccer match that I attended between my favourite team Watford, playing Liverpool in a cup match. Two family friends were going to the game and I asked them if they would give me a lift as they were Watford followers as well.

I walked to their apartment to meet with them and then we drove to the game. One asked me, "where would I be standing?" I told them, "I would be standing in the Vicarage Road end." Arriving at the stadium in plenty of time, we had a bit of a wait before kickoff and my friends would be sitting in another part of the stadium. We parted and I told them that I would meet them after the game in the stadium.

When getting to the place where I would be standing, there were hardly any fans there and I got to stand in the very front. As more fans started arriving, it looked like it was going to be a big crowd tonight.

When the referee led the two teams out onto the pitch, cheers from the fans of both sides started to fill the air. I was excited, just as much as everyone else was. Where I was standing which was at the front of the crowd and a brick wall in front of me, now it was a tight squeeze, as that end was completely filled with fans.

Watford kicked off and started well. After 15 minutes into the game and I was in need of going to the toilet, but as I was tight against a wall, I could hardly move. Later in the first half Watford had a free kick, just outside the penalty box and they were kicking towards my end of the ground. The Watford fans held their breath as the ball sailed into the area and into the back of the net.

GOAL! Watford had scored and the fans went wild including me!

Liverpool kicked off again and the excitement in the air was electrifying. A few moments later, I started to get a taste in my mouth and starting to have a partial seizure. This went on a few seconds then unfortunately went into a major seizure and I was in trouble. OH NO!

Fans standing around me could see that I was in trouble and that I was shaking, so they shouted for the stewards to come over. Two of them raced over and dragged me out of the crowd and took me along the side of the pitch to the other end of the ground. They took me passed the part where my friends were sitting and they looked on and saw me dragged along and still having a seizure. I was taken to the First Aid room and laid on a day bed. "Are you OK?" Asked one of the first aiders. By then the seizure had stopped and could answer them "I am OK."

During Half time, one of my friends came to the First Aid room to see me. He asked, "If I was, OK?" I replied "Yes I was." However, I was not going to be able to go back and see the rest of the game. "Too bad, we will come by after the game and take you back home." "OK then," I said.

My friend left and returned to his seat and the second half began. All of a sudden, there was a big roar as if a goal had been scored and somebody popped their head in to say that Liverpool had scored a goal making it 1 – 1 in the closing stages of the second half.

To my disappointment, I was going to spend the rest of the game in the First Aid room. The game went into extra time in which Liverpool scored a second goal and Watford lost 1-2.

After the final whistle, my friends came for me and we all made our way back to the car to go home.

What a night? Having a seizure during the game and my team lost. Surely something that was not planned for me, nor for them.

Hopefully there would be no more occasions like that during games.

Watford Stadium
My File photo

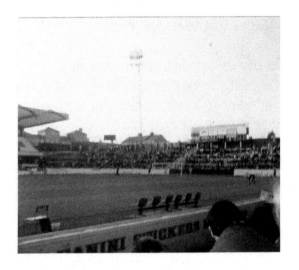

Starting Life on My Own

Still living with my parents in 1989, the situation in the household was a little stressful for all of us. We were having regular arguments during the weekends over all sorts of small matters, nothing serious or abusive, but shouting and yelling at each other.

My dad complained a lot and I had arguments with my mother. My sister and I did not get on, as she is a bit of a rebel of doing things her way and there was no stopping her, even if she was in the wrong. It was time to get out and get some independence for myself.

A member of the local authority from the housing department came to my parent's house on one occasion and classed my parent's place as overcrowded, as there were five of us living there.

Despite my epilepsy, I decided to apply to the local authority and put my name on the housing list of tenants to have a place of my own.

A year had gone by since that visit by the local authority with no offers.

Then after eighteen months of waiting, in 1991 a letter arrived. The postman brought the letter that I had been waiting for. There was an apartment available that we could go and take a look at, as it was empty and ready for someone to move into.

What a surprise! An offer from the local authority. It was a place only half a mile away from my parent's home. This was hopefully to be my new start.

An appointment was arranged to meet with a lady from the local authority at the apartment that could possibly be mine. We met and the lady unlocked the door and walked in first. It had one large room that was a bedroom and living room combination with a large window and a reasonable size kitchen off it plus a small bathroom.

As I was being shown the apartment, my feelings grew happier with what I was seeing, thinking that this place could be mine. After the viewing, I said without hesitation to her that I would take it.

After waiting for eighteen months, I was not going to let the epilepsy stop me from having my independence and living on my own.

On my birthday, I received the best present, of the keys to the apartment and so a fresh new start in my life's journey.

Between the months of July and September, I was regularly cleaning and sweeping the apartment and my dad helped to decorate it with me and make it feel like home. Family and friends were kind enough to give me items that were needed to start this new life.

They knew that I virtually had nothing to start a life on my own with all the items needed to do so. With their help and love, they gave me furniture which included: a bed, carpet, sofa and a kettle. The only things I had to bring that were mine were items from my bedroom at my parent's home.

My mother was understandably worried about me having seizures while living in the apartment alone. When September arrived, I moved into the apartment and hoped that in time my mother would see that I would be alright.

Getting along with the neighbours was fine, but most of the time, I kept to myself in the communal living area. But there was one unfortunate occasion, when I had a seizure right outside the apartments, where the garages were, and some of the neighbours unfortunately saw this happen.

One of my neighbours who was aware of my epilepsy, helped me through it by putting a coat under my head, so that I would not swallow my tongue. It was later on that day that he told me what had happened as I did not know what had happened during the seizure.

Overall, I settled in nicely living on my own. It was much quieter, compared to what it was like some of the times living with my mother, dad and siblings. I ended up living at this apartment for 20 years before managing to acquire a one-bedroom apartment.

Training for Work

After leaving school, I went onto a Youth Training Scheme (YTS) programme at the West Herts College in Hemel Hempstead from 1985 to 1986.

However, I was restricted to the type of work that I could apply for as in working on machinery for obvious reasons or on a computer due to the flashes from the monitor screen that may bring on a seizure. What it meant was that I could have any type of job that I liked that did not involve those things.

While on the YTS programme, we had lessons at the Dacorum College that could be work related, as in practising typing skills in which my typing speed was not very good and also written work that we were given to do.

Unfortunately, on different occasions in the classroom, I had seizures and the person in charge of the class would do what was needed to be done to help me get through the seizure as safely as possible.

At times during lunch breaks, there were different activities in the gym hall. The times I enjoyed most was when there were one hour trampoline sessions. I would be connected to a harness and would do things such as jumping up and down plus somersaults and landing on my feet. The time always felt very short for others who were in line to do the same thing and having their turn.

After a few weeks, those on the YTS programme started their work placements, in hope of securing a job there in time.

I started working at the Dacorum Pavilion for a few weeks, which involved things like emptying bottles, such as coke and beer bottles etc. and place back in their crates or to be thrown away as some were broken, having to be very careful not to cut my fingers open.

Also cleaning up and setting out tables and chairs for a function or a performance on the stage. They needed chairs to be set out, two wide long rows going from the stage to the back of the hall. Then the following morning after the entertainment, the chairs needed to be put away.

On one occasion, a wrestling event was taking place. I and other workers placed a large wrestling ring in the centre of the main hall and then placed seating around all four sides of the ring. The chairs were fold up types, making it pretty easy to do.

As I was doing a good job, the manager of the Pavilion called me to his office. He asked me if I would like to have a complementary ticket to the event. This I accepted and was very excited to be able to watch the Professional Wrestling matches.

I told him that I was a wrestling fan and watched it on TV on a Saturday afternoon and thanking him for this opportunity. I am sure he could see it written all over my face.

It would give me the chance to see Giant Haystacks fight plus others for real.

It was a great occasion as when the evening came, my seat was very close to the ring and where the wrestlers walked out from their dressing rooms, they walked pass me close up. I had a great night, what a treat.

However; despite the fact that I enjoyed working there, sadly a permanent job was not in the offering for me.

Another placement that came along that I could try was at the local Co-Op Express Dairy at the back of the Hemel Hempstead town centre. I would arrive there about 7:30 am and report to the gentleman in charge.

The job that I had would involve cleaning the yard out, including sweeping the delivery area where the trucks would be parked and spraying water on the floor to wash away any milk, through milk bottles falling off the delivery trucks or being dropped.

One morning, I woke up very early and decided to go into the Co-Op dairy at 4:30 am, as the milkmen would be there loading their delivery trucks to do their rounds. As a result of arriving early, I was allowed to go out on a milk round with one of the milkmen.

Bill was his name and off we went to do his rounds. Heading around the roads in town and when we came to an apartment that he had orders for, Bill let me take the milk to it and collect the empty bottles that were left out the night before.

Sometimes, they had a note at the top of the milk bottle saying no milk today, or asking for eggs or something else that was carried on the delivery truck.

Depending on the note, I would follow the instructions. Taking the order down of what was wanted. This was something new for me and I enjoyed doing it. When we completed the round, Bill drove back to the yard.

At the end of my two weeks there despite how well I worked, they had no vacancies available unfortunately, so once again nothing materialized.

I continued on at the Youth Training Scheme programme for the twelve months that the training sessions went on for. But by the end of the Youth Training Scheme, I had no luck in finding a job and had to try something else.

1986 Garston Manor

Having no success on the Youth Training Scheme, my next step towards finding work was to take a course at Garston Manor. Garston Manor was a place that helped people with difficulties to find work. I hoped that it would work for me also.

I started the program in August and settled into the program just fine. The type of work and teachings provided, included finding out what I would be good at and what I would not do well with. Some of the workshops involved measuring, marking out the measurements then cutting exercises plus more. This proved to be difficult for me in coping with these methods.

Basic geometry was poor, and I was restricted to doing certain things due to the risks of having a seizure. I was given a mark of (C) for standard and the same for speed when doing the tests.

Another test involved the use of a Meccano set. An assembling exercise using perforated metal parts. My performance showed that I had difficulty in recognizing the location and shapes. Receiving a (B) mark for that, which was standard, however I was rather slow with how long it took me to complete the task at thirty-eight minutes. They gave me a (D) mark for speed.

On the circuit testing exercise, I made two errors and it took me eighty minutes to complete. The mark was a (B) for standard and a poor (E) mark for speed.

During the time of doing the course there was on one occasion while sitting down, I had a seizure which went virtually unrecognized.

Next, I was tested on a nuts & bolts assembly and once again had restricted access due to the dangers of a possible seizure.

Did not do bad on it though, scoring an (A) mark for standard and (B) for speed. It appeared that I was better using larger components and less decision-making being involved.

Other exercises included installing computer programmes in which I coped quite easily having a computer at home called a ZX81. Making a few errors, I was able to quickly correct them without any help.

Other skills included basic mathematics, receiving 60%, I felt positive about that.

The overall summery of tasks completed led to a report saying that 'Peter put a very good effort in throughout the testing. The most promising performance being shown on a set of straight forward semi clerical exercises. His job prospects however are not too encouraging at this time; however, this position should greatly improve if the frequency of his seizures could be diminished and his GP (doctor) has suggested treatment at the Chalfont Centre for Epilepsy.'

A Stay at the Chalfont Centre

After I finished at Garston Manor, my doctor made arrangements for me to attend a place for people with epilepsy called The Chalfont Centre for Epilepsy.

Having already had epilepsy for seventeen years and no real breakthrough in sorting out the health issue, my consultant who I was under for the epilepsy was called Professor Simon Shorvon.

The time was going to be from September to December 1987. My parent's and I were happy about doing this, for they could come and see me on the weekends or since I was living reasonably close to the Centre, I could go home to them.

This was the next attempt at trying to get me onto the right medication to better control the seizures that was currently not working all that well.

When September came along, my dad and mother took me to the Chalfont Centre for

Epilepsy to begin the assessment programme. I was taking Tegretol of 300mg in the morning and 200mg in the evening. Also, I was taking Sodium Valproate 1 gram, 2 tablets a day at that time.

Upon arriving we went to the reception area to report in. I was then taken to the house that I would be staying in, along with other males of different ages. The name of the house was Susan Edwards.

After being introduced to the staff, I was shown where my cubicle was, as in my bed area. Just like a hospital ward really where everybody's cubicle was next to each other.

As my parent's decided to make a move to go back home, I gave them a hug and we said our goodbyes before they left.

Afterwards, I went to join the rest of the people who were staying in the same house and introduced ourselves.

In the evening of my first day, I saw a person have a seizure in the lounge.

I don't know if he had some kind of warning like I do with mine, as a taste in the mouth. He started to take some of his clothes off while in the seizure and I thought before arriving at the centre that the type of seizures that I had was the only type there was.

I had never seen a person having an epileptic seizure until now. This was very surprising for me to see that there were other types. When the others saw him start to have a seizure, they called for the staff's attention.

The lady on duty came and laid him on the ground and waited for him to come out of his seizure. When he did, he put his clothes back on and was taken to his cubicle bedroom.

Overall, I settled in fine and eventually when it was time to, I went to bed and slept OK on my first night there. It did seem weird by not being in my own bed.

Next morning of my first full day, I was taken around the centre and shown where different activities were done, such as artwork, writing for the centre magazine which went around every week. They also showed me where the other houses were.

Amongst the activities that the patients could do during the week would be an optional exercise class that happened once a day. This was of great interest to me and joined in whenever I could. The exercises focused on balancing your body and requiring stable movements. At the end, we finished the exercise session by laying on the floor for about four minutes while relaxing from the energy that had been used.

I enjoyed it very much and it was well attended by other individuals who lived at the centre.

Another activity that was very enjoyable was being taken to the local swimming baths once a week. There were seven to ten people from the centre each week that would go swimming. This activity was great to do as it was a time to get away from the centre and enjoy the water.

The lady that took us was in her thirties and a very nice person. When we would go, I would always get very excited, looking forward to swimming as we climbed into the mini bus and were driven to the pool.

After arriving, we went to the changing rooms, changing into our trunks and off into the pool. This was the start of having lots of fun in the water and getting the exercise by doing lengths of the pool. There was also a diving board that I loved to use.

Unfortunately, on some occasions, while swimming, I witnessed people having seizures while in the pool, getting dragged out by the life guard and taken back to the changing rooms. I felt shaken whenever I saw this happen and felt sorry for the person who had the seizure.

Loving to write, I started to write a feature in the magazine that was produced for the centre in the Art Room, and began a little story called 'The Joker,' about how I dived into the pool when going swimming, doing drawings of me diving to go with the story and creating a plot about a certain person which was me. That I had an eye on a staff member, who was the lady that took us to the swimming baths each week, writing a small piece for the magazine each week.

As the weeks went by, people were coming up to me asking me who this person was, but I did not say anything. It was fun to do, keeping people guessing. However, in the end, it did come out of who it was. Glad that the staff member concerned did not mind.

Back at the Susan Edwards House, due to a rota procedure, we would be taking turns doing such tasks as washing up, drying up after meal times, cleaning and other tasks. I felt OK about doing these tasks and just did them when it was my turn. None of us complained about it and we did our jobs.

During October, the person that arranged events for people to go to or do had acquired a few tickets for a European Qualifier Soccer match at Wembley Stadium in London between England and Turkey on the 14th of October. As there were only a few tickets, only a few people would be able to attend the match.

Fortunately, I was one of the lucky ones picked to go.

I was very excited to be going, as I had never been to Wembley Stadium before nor had seen England play and this made me very, very happy indeed.

When the day came of the soccer match, those going went and got ready to go. The lucky people going to the match walked to where the mini bus was parked and waited for the lady to arrive and take us there. When she did, we were on our way to Wembley Stadium. It was a wet rainy evening. We were all very excited, talking and smiling to each other while looking forward to getting there and the game to start.

Eventually arriving in London, the lady parked the minibus and we all got out. I could not get out quickly enough as I was feeling that excited to finally be there. We walked to the stadium to find there was a long line of people waiting outside to get in. So, we joined the long queue of England fans standing in the rain. To our disappointment we had arrived a bit late and were still in the queue outside the stadium when the soccer match started.

We moved through the turnstiles with her handing all the tickets to the man at the gate, we then made our way to our seats.

By then, England had already scored two goals and were winning 2-0 when we eventually got to our seats. I was feeling a bit frustrated, but I thought to myself that the delay in the queue could not have been helped.

England played very well in the first half and we were chanting "Come on England," cheering the team on waving our scarves and when they scored a third goal, I jumped for joy with sheer excitement along with the others.

The atmosphere in the stadium was electric. By half time England was winning 4-0. However, the heavy rain was still coming down.

During half time, some of us had a hot drink to keep warm or something to eat and also talked about how good the first half was.

The teams came out for the second half and England carried on playing the same way they had been doing at the end of the first half, and looking like more goals would come. They had a few chances to score and each time we stood up and said to each other "Nearly a goal." It was not that long before England did score a fifth goal in the 59th minute.

We could not have been happier to see England play, this was very enjoyable indeed. A sixth goal was scored and we were certainly now thrashing the Turkey soccer team.

Another goal was scored to make it 7-0 and England even had time to score another goal. We were all very happy as the referee blew the final whistle and celebrated an 8-0 win for the home team.

We started to make our way, walking out of the stadium and I was feeling very chirpy with myself along with the other forty-five and a half thousand people that attended the match. The rain did not dampen the mood and being dripping wet was overshadowed by the great win for England.

Reaching the mini bus, everyone got in and we were driven back to the centre, arriving very late indeed. Everyone was dropped off at the homes they were staying at. It had been a very good nights event, despite the wet conditions throughout the evening.

The very next evening, the wind started to pick up and was getting stronger when we went to bed. It was a bit frightening to say the least. There was lots of rain and wind lashing against the windows by our beds. We could hear the trees being blown around. Through all that, I did get to sleep and slept through it, while others struggled to sleep, so they got up and went into the lounge and watched some television.

In the morning, I woke up like the other lads and looked out the window and was in shock and horror to see branches all over the ground that had broken off the trees.

After breakfast, we went outside to take a look around the grounds and were met with the sight of carnage around the centre. As we made our way to the other end of the centre where the workshops were, I thought to myself "GOSH," looking in horror at a large tall tree that had been blown out of the ground during the night and landed on the roof of one of the other houses.

It seemed that the patients and staff living in that house were moved out and taken to another house.

People went round and gave a hand in tidying the grounds up and taking some of the large branches to the workshop, where they would be cut up into logs. I was thinking blimey, a lot of trees had been damaged.

The local TV news channel would be coming to report on what had happened at the centre along with other areas affected. They arrived and filmed the areas damaged the most and also some of us in the workshop cutting the logs up into small sized ones, as there was no need to waste the wood as it would come in handy.

When we watched the evening news, it showed the damage of the centre. They also reported on the people working in the workshop. In which I saw the back of myself on the television and pointed to the television saying, "look, there I am."

We could not believe that the weather could do such damage and the weather forecasters did not say anything about it coming before the event happened either.

Another time after having a blood test done, I had an appointment with the doctor and it was decided to take me off the Sodium Valproate and increase my Tegretol to 600 mgs in the morning and 600 mgs in the evening. Hopefully this was going to make a difference for me in time.

Being taken off the Sodium Valproate did cause me to continue having seizures though and I had some major seizures, having three in one day. Despite the fact that people staying at the Susan Edwards House saw me have seizures, I never asked or was told what I did during an episode, and I was none the wiser on that front.

One day, a few of us went to a local sports centre to play a few games of five-a-side soccer. The teams were picked by the supervisor at the sports centre. The team I played for, I was placed in the goal to be the goalkeeper. So, when our first game arrived, all the players playing were eager to play and the game kicked off.

During the game, I was standing in goal as the action was at the other end, when all of a sudden, my right leg gave way on me, losing my balance and I fell backwards and landed on my bum. Totally in shock and wondered what had happened.

The staff member who brought us to the sports centre came over to me and asked me if I was OK, as I had not gotten up yet. I told them that my knee just went out on me while I was just standing.

"It looks as if we may need to take you to the hospital," the staff member said. What the hell has happened to me?

I was taken from the Sports centre to a nearby Hospital by the staff member. Arriving at the hospital and went to the Accident & Emergency department and waited. Still in shock and worried about what had happened to my leg.

When I was eventually called in by the nurse and had the leg x-rayed, the doctor came and looked at the x-ray. He saw there was some damage to the ligament and told me that we will have to put a plaster cast on the leg.

OH NO! I thought to myself, quite stunned to hear this. What a night this is turning out to be! I was escorted to the plaster room and when I sat down, the nurse started to plaster my leg up from near the top of my leg down to just above my ankle. I was given crutches to use. Once done, I left the plaster room. We made our way out of the hospital and back to the centre.

Despite the fact that I was in plaster, it did not stop me attempting doing the exercise classes that took place daily. Though, perhaps I should not have been doing them. The music used was the whole of the George Michael album 'Faith'. It was a great motivation for me to exercise with.

Attempted to do them, but lost my balance and fell over while doing the standing ones. I decided that it would be best for me to take a break from going to the class due to damaging not just the plaster but also not doing my knee any good either.

Eventually, after about a week or two of hobbling around, the plaster was removed and glad it was, as I had been missing the swimming and many other activities.

One evening at the Susan Edwards house, I was sitting in the dining room, just after we had finished our tea. Another person was standing at the sink washing up the plates, cutlery etc, when out of the blue, he started to have a seizure and collapsed falling backwards.

There was a dining table behind him where I was sitting and he banged the back of his head onto the table as he fell backwards towards the ground.

He was a tall and well-built gentleman and he went down hard. I was shocked at seeing this and shouted out for the house master on duty, who came rushing into the kitchen and placed a few tea towels rolled up under his head so that he did not swallow his tongue, until he came out of his seizure.

Some of the other lads came in, but were told, including myself to go back into the lounge, while the unfortunate man was being seen to.

He came round OK, but was told to go and lay down on his bed after taking a nasty whack on the back of his head.

Another evening, a few of us decided to go out for the evening and take a walk into the town centre, which was half a mile away. This was something that we were allowed to do. We made our way towards town, feeling very happy to be having a night out.

Arriving in town about 7 pm and finding a pub, we strolled through the door. Went to the bar, I ordered a 'Shandy' *(pint of ½ lager and ½ lemonade)* once everyone was served, we decided to go and play a game of darts. Two of us started to play, while the others stood and watched as they chatted and enjoyed the time out.

Sitting near us were two men and a woman at a table close to the entrance of the pub. All of a sudden, an argument broke out between the two gentleman and we stood in disbelief.

One of the men started shouting at the other gentleman in a rage for whatever reason. He did get himself into a bad temper while the lady looked on at him in an annoying way. She appeared to be embarrassed seeing her friend act in such a way plus seeing everyone in the pub watching on.

After a few minutes of his temper going on, he picked up the chair that he was sitting on and as he did, the lady moved off her seat in such a rush to get out of the way as she looked very frightened. With a quick move he threw it at the pub's glass window and the chair went smashing through it.

The glass shattered and made a lot of noise. He shouted a few more words in anger then headed towards the exit of the pub and stormed out. The lady was upset and started to cry.

The owner of the pub came over to the other two and asked them to leave the pub without any hesitation. They tried to back themselves up acting innocent saying that it was the fault of the one that had smashed the glass, but with no luck, they walked out the pub together.

We all just stood there in shock and amazed as to what had happened. Not believing what we had just witnessed. "I wonder what that was about?" I said to one of the others, one replied "search me."

Moments later, after we gain our wits back, the game of darts started once again. Shortly after that, one of the lads from our group started to have a seizure and started shaking. He fell to the ground and landed with a bump.

We turned and saw him fall to the ground, but not quick enough for any of us to catch him.

We went over to help him. He was put on his side and a coat was put under his head.

Eventually, he stopped shaking and came out of the seizure. He rested on the floor for a few moments, until he felt ready to get up, then we helped him up and sat him down on a bench near us. "Is he OK over there?" Someone nearby asked. Someone replied; "Yes he is with us, thanks."

"What a night this was turning out to be?" I said. "Yes," they replied and around 10:30 pm, we decided to make our way back to the centre.

We were talking about the events of the evening in the pub. "Boy! We were not expecting an evening filled with that much excitement and drama behind it all?" Someone said. With that the group agreed and we walked towards our house. "Good night," I said to all.

Once in bed, the events of the evening played over and over in my head until I finally went to sleep.

One evening a week, a few of us were taken out the centre and went to a local P.H.A.B club, *(P.H.A.B stands for Physically, Handicap and Body)* in which you could do different activities like play table tennis, pool and make friends with others from different locations.

The second week that I went there, I started talking to a woman who went there also, her name was Mandy. I saw her when arriving at the club and took it upon myself to go over and say hello. We talked to each other about many things and at times had a good laugh about some of the stories we told of the different events that we did. It was enjoyable talking with her and I did like her even though it was only going to be at the P.H.A.B that we would meet.

From then onwards, we became very good friends. After I finished at the centre in December 1987, we wrote letters to each other as friends for a while until things faded away and Mandy stopped writing. I thought it was a shame, for we did get on well.

December came, and I had done the three months at the centre, so it was going to be time to leave and go back home. When that day came, I got my things packed up and my parents came for me. I went around and thanked the staff before leaving Susan Edwards House for the last time and told them that I enjoyed my stay.

Unfortunately, I left the centre with no real breakthrough on the medical side, and continued to have major seizures.

What a time it had been while staying at the centre. With the unexpected surprise of seeing that there was more than my own type of seizures.

Then having my leg in a plaster, which was not a good thing at all, stopping me for a time in doing such activities like badminton, swimming and the exercise class that I loved to do.

Having many different life experiences and learning a lot during my time there. Seemed to me I was growing up in many ways. Seeing what can happen from a nasty storm and the nasty incident at the pub.

Most of all, I found great pleasure in making new friends and the outings we would go on our own are great memories for me. Those times we went out with the staff member, taking us to different events was a treat and a nice change from daily life at the centre.

It was there that I found out that I really enjoyed writing for the centre's newsletter, thus showing that I had some creativity towards writing, yet was not aware of at that time.

Aiming for a Better Life

In 1988, I joined the local job club and went twice a week. We had to send out 10 letters that included a Resume/CV.

I would spend many hours writing letters and sending them out that matched my key skills to businesses that were advertising jobs or just sending spec letters. However, for one reason or another, including having the epilepsy, I was being turned down.

One day an interview came up at St Paul's Hospital. They were advertising a Porter's position that I applied for. When I attended the interview, I had three members of management sitting in front of me in which one was the manager of the Portering Department.

Needless to say, as I sat in front of them my nervousness kicked in as they started to ask questions to me relating to my fitness and they also addressed my situation relating to the epilepsy, happy that they were aware of it.

They actually had two job positions to offer me of a general porter or a garbage/laundry porter. I decided to go for the garbage/laundry porter's job.

After the job interview was over, they said that they would let me know in due course as they had other people to interview. I left the office and went home, feeling that we got along well and everything was out in the open. Now it was time to just sit and wait to hear if the job was mine or not.

Success came as a letter arrived through the post to tell me that I had the job and would I like to start in May 1988, my reply was a resounding yes.

The position was a basic job of collecting bags of garbage and waste food bags from the hospital wards, plus any bags of garbage from other departments around the hospital. To do this, I used a cart to collect it all in.

For part of the day, I also would work in the linen department, helping out with delivering the clean linen to the wards and bringing back the dirty linen.

Pushing the cart to the different hospital wards was difficult at times, because from the linen room to the wards it was uphill and depending on how much laundry was on the cart making it heavier, then it would be more difficult to push. Then during the winter months when snow was on the ground that had not been shovelled, made matters worse.

At some point during the day, the dirty linen was picked up by a laundry company based in London, washed and brought back to the linen room to be sorted and placed onto the cart for delivery.

In 1993, St Paul's Hospital was closed down and the doctors, nurses and staff members were transferred to a much larger hospital in the same town called the West Herts Hospital.

Where I was doing virtually the same job as before, except on a much larger scale. As for my epilepsy, I had a few major incidents at work over my time there, however they were pretty bad ones.

The first time, I was at the back of the hospital emptying a cart load of garbage, when I had a seizure and banged the back of my head onto a sharp bit of metal, cutting my head open AGAIN! Somehow though, I managed to walk from the back of the hospital to the front entrance and into the emergency department without knowing how I got there, as I was so dazed.

On a regular basis, I was being sent home after having seizures and being taken to the emergency department.

Another major incident involving my seizures happened in 1994, outside the Verulam

Wing. "This was to be the last straw," said the manager of the Personnel Department.

In 1995, I was laid off/suspended for medical reasons for a year, which seemed unfair, since they did know of my condition at the hospital when they first hired me.

Deciding that I needed some advice, I went to the Citizen Advice Bureau, where I met with Mr. Bond.

After discussing the situation with Mr. Bond, he decided to attend the meetings with me between myself and the Personnel Department of the hospital.

Despite the money being offered to me by the hospital, it was my intention to take them to a Tribunal. If it was not for Mr. Bond attending these meetings with me, the hospital would have gotten away with paying less than they had intended to in the end. The whole issue was finalized in 1996 when they paid up out of court.

What I Had Done and not Done Up to October 1996

Had Done

1. I was living on my own
2. I had gained some independence
3. I had played soccer for a local Pub

My Dreams

1. Going on vacation/holiday abroad
2. My epilepsy to be improved
3. Travelling on long journeys
4. Doing things in public
   (Karaoke and in competitions)
5. Gain more confidence
6. Learn to use computers without the fear of having seizures
7. Learn to drive a car
8. Working on machinery

Decision Time

Over time, since I started having the epilepsy, doctor's have been making the decisions on taking me off or putting me on different types of medications, as they either were not working or mixing well with the other tablets that I was taking at that time, and there were some that did not mix with the Tegretol, as that was the medication that I have taken most of my life to date.

Over the years, since the start of the epilepsy, I have used the medications including Tegretol, Frisium, Phenytoin, Ospolot, Diazepam, Valproate, Epilim and Gabapentin.

During 1995, it was decided to put me onto another medication called Lamictal. It was virtually one of the last ones that were available for me to try with all the medications that I have tried over the years (as above), since I first began taking medication, trying to keep the seizures down. I was having between 55 and 69 major seizures every year.

In May of 1995, I had an appointment at the National Hospital for Neurosurgery and Neurology to see my consultant Professor Simon Shorvon.

My dad attended the appointment with me. We were in the waiting room for a while when my dad started moaning about how long it was taking for them to call me in. Finally, my name was called out. "About time too," my dad said. So, we made our way to the consultant room. "Hello Peter," Professor Shorvon said, as we entered the room. "Come in and sit down."

After asking me how things had been going, relating to the epilepsy, and I told him my story, he said; "There was one last chance available to possibly sort your epilepsy out."

"There is a new M.R.I. (Magnetic Resonance Imaging) scanning machine being placed in the Chalfont Centre for Epilepsy," he told us that the new M.R.I. would be ready for operation soon.

At this time, the M.R.I was the latest in this technology to date. This scanning machine could view the inside of the brain and the possibility of finding the issues that were causing the seizures to start with, plus view what damage there was inside the brain.

He asked me, if I would like him to put my name forward to have a scan done to see if anything could be found. My reply was "OK then."

He said that he would send a letter to the Chalfont Centre for Epilepsy to get my name on the list. With that, we stood up and said our goodbyes to the Professor and left the room to make our way home.

A few weeks later, I received a letter through the mail from the Chalfont Centre for Epilepsy, with an appointment date of January 1996 to attend the centre and have a scan done.

In January 1996, I made my way to have the M.R.I. scan with both parent's taking me there. "I wonder if anything was going to be found?" I said to them. Mother was very hopeful, "Let's hope so, with all the other tests that you have had over the years, and nothing found."

With that, I thought positively about the M.R.I. scan being done, and that something good would come from that.

We arrive at the centre and dad parked the car and we all went to the reception area to book in.

While in the waiting room, a nurse came up to me and said; "You will need to take your watch off and any other items that you have to do with metal, such as coins, as that could affect the machine working properly."

I took the certain items off and any lose change out of my pocket.

A few minutes later, the same nurse said from the door where the M.R.I machine was that "We are ready for you now, would you like to come through." I was asked to please take my shoes off. Then I was told to lay down on the table.

Laying flat on the table (just like on an x-ray machine), they gave me earplugs to wear as the machine would make a loud noise or bangs during the tests.

As I lay there, as still as I could, every so often while they were taking scans, I heard the loud noises, but could not see what was being done. After three scans were taken, I was brought back out of the tunnel and was told that all had been done.

Arriving back to my parents in the waiting room, I asked the nurse, "Any chance of getting the results today?" The nurse replied; "You won't be getting them today. They will be sent back to your consultant." I would have to wait for the scan results until my next appointment.

When my next appointment with Professor Shorvon came, he gave me the results of the scans. "The tests show that there is residual scar tissue on the lefthand side of the brain; which had never been discovered before, even though it had probably been there since the start of the epilepsy, when during the time of having convulsions, the blood would have been shooting up into the brain."

He also said "The scarring having been found on the lefthand side of the brain, there could be a chance of having an operation, which may be your last chance saloon for you to find relief from the epilepsy." "We will need to have a couple of tests done at The National Hospital for Neurosurgery/Neurology in London to be carried out first, and both tests would have to show positive results to possibly give you the chance to have the operation."

"OK then, I will go along with that and see what happens."

So, when Monday July 15 1996 came along, and I packed my clothes up and the other things that I would require. My parent's drove me to London to the National Hospital for Neurosurgery and Neurology to have the first of the two tests done.

It was going to be a five day stay in the hospital from the 15th to the 19th July for the first part of the testing.

We were told to be there early in keeping with the appointment, so we arrived at 8:30 am and walked into the hospital, reporting to the reception desk.

A few moments later, someone came along to take us to the ward. When we arrived there, I was taken to a cubicle and by the bedside there was a machine that I would be connected up to by a cable. Also, a monitor (CCTV) was on the wall pointed directly to the bed. They were going to be watching me all the time for if a seizure would occur, it could be recorded.

Once settled in, my parent's said goodbye to me and left the ward and headed home.

The consultant that I was going to be under during my stay at the hospital was a gentleman called Mr. Fish.

After changing into my pyjamas and dressing gown, a nurse came along and connected the wires to my head using sticky black round sucker things.

Prolonged monitoring was going to be starting at 11 am that same day and carry on till my final day when I would go home.

The first things they did was to lower my dosage of medications. This was done so that seizures would happen.

The Tegretol was reduced to 200 mgs in the morning and 150 mgs in the evening and the Lactimal was reduced to 25 mgs for both morning and evening. Gabapentin would be reduced to 200 mgs and finally the Clobazam would remain at 10 mg. Within a day after the reduction of the medications, seizures started to happen.

On the 17th of July, I had a total of five seizures through the day. They were all stereotyped. Getting a taste in the mouth before each seizure, which I had always thought was a warning before each one happened, when actually it was a partial seizure that led into a full-blown seizure on occasions.

When having each seizure, which was seen by the staff on duty via the video camera, they saw what I did, first came fidgety movements for the first 13 to 26 seconds, such as moving my head, folding my arms around my stomach and shifting of body position and also touching my face.

My left hand in all cases of the seizures started repeatedly to be wiping my face. The right arm remained stiff for between twenty-five and forty-four seconds.

The fidgeting slowly ceases and I could not talk properly for around three minutes after a major seizure happened.

Sometimes after the seizure, I felt tired and would fall to sleep.

On one occasion, I was sitting at the side of the bed in the cubicle, when one of the seizures happened and the nurse rushed from the nurse's station as a monitor was on at all times and someone was always watching. This was to make sure that patients did not hurt themselves if falling to the floor.

They put me in a safe position of laying me onto the bed until I came around.

Next day, my parents came to visit me. "Hello," my mother said, giving me a cuddle. "Hi mother."

They sat down beside the bed. "We came to see how you were doing." They both could see that I was happy and doing fine. They brought me in a bag of sweets, just like my mother use to send to me by mail, when I was at the boarding school in Torquay.

We continued chatting, while I lay on the bed wired up to the equipment. I told them that the seizures had started to happen now and the Doctors and Nurses will be gathering up the evidence. They also watch when they happen, keeping notes on whatever it is that I do during a seizure.

The tea lady came round while my parent's were there and we were asked if we would like a cup of tea and we all said; "yes please."

"How was everyone at home?" And dad replied; "everyone is OK."

When we had finished our tea, my parent's decided that they were going to set off for home. Both gave me hugs, and said their goodbyes.

Not long after they had gone, a member of staff came to me and asked if I could come with her. First, she had to take the cables off the machine and then I was able to walk to another part of the ward with them. The room was where items such as toys and activities were done for testing the patients.

I was asked to perform tasks in which they were going to test the brain on how fast or slow it reacted to doing a particular task at hand, as in naming an item or doing something with objects.

Some were easy to do and some were hard. Such as picking up a ball which was fine or drawing a tree that was not a bad effort, but obviously they were looking at how the brain was reacting to the messages given. I spent about half an hour doing these tasks then I was led back to my cubicle.

Not long after returning, another seizure started. Once again, a staff member rushed over to the cubicle, as I was sitting on the side of the bed and they arrived before I slid off it and possibly may have hit the floor hurting myself. I was held during the seizure while sitting on the side of the bed. Before being placed back onto the bed after the seizure had finished.

On the Wednesday, I was reading books and soccer magazines in bed when my doctor arrived. He stood beside the bed and said, "Morning Peter." I replied "Hello Doctor."

Taking a look at the notes that he was holding, he said to me, "Your seizures are triggering from the lefthand side of the brain and due to that, there is a possibility that we could move forward towards thinking of an operation." My Reply was "That would be good then."

"How well are you feeling?" He asked me. "I am feeling fine."

"Your medication will be going back up to their normal levels tomorrow," he said and with that he walked off to his next patient.

Later that day, I did some more tests in a room elsewhere in the ward and after that it was a bit of a quiet day that followed.

During that same day, my mother and dad also arrived to visit me. I told them about all that had been going on, the tests results and about the seizures. Also, that the Doctor said it may be possible for an operation. Plus, I would be able to go home tomorrow. They were both very happy about the results. Mother then said that "Dad would come back and pick me up tomorrow."

Dad said "We cannot stay long as we have someone coming this evening." With that, they started walking and mother turns with a smile and says "See you tomorrow, Peter."

On the Friday morning, after having breakfast, the nurse came to disconnect me from the monitor. It was then that I asked her, "Is it possible to see one of the seizures I had that was filmed?" Telling her that I had never known or been told what happened to me during a seizure. The nurse replied "I will go and see about that for you," and off she went.

I started to pack everything, to be ready for dad, when he would arrive to take me home.

Nearly packed and dressed when the nurse came back in; "Peter, it is possible for you to see one of your seizures." "Good then," I replied.

Just then, dad arrived at the cubicle. "Morning son." I replied "Hi Dad," and as I did, the monitor screen on the wall came on and started to show one of my seizures that I had earlier in the week.

'I was laying in bed sitting up and started twitching, then folding my arms over my stomach, I lifted my left arm up to my face and started wiping my face in a motion from the forehead down to my chin, while the right arm remained stiff for twenty to thirty seconds. I started to drool as my left arm went back down into the folding position. Overall, the seizure lasted about two to three minutes.'

After watching the monitor, it took a few moments to digest it all. But at least I now knew what happens and perhaps I would be able to explain it more to my GP, as to what actually happens during an episode.

Turning my attention back to getting ready and packed the rest of my belongings.

Time to leave, so we passed the nursing station, I stopped and said, "Thank you for all the caring and help you gave to me." The Doctor happened to be there and I reached out and shook the Doctors hand. They knew that with the possibility of improvement to my issues, my life could change for the better in time.

Leaving the ward with my dad, we walked towards the entrance of the hospital to where dad had parked his car. It felt good to be heading back home. Dad dropped me off at my apartment. "Thank you, dad, for the lift and tell mother that I will call her later, Bye."

Now back in my own apartment and back home, I sat down and thought about everything that happened over the past few days. Part of me was very happy to know that if I passed the next set of tests, then I could have the surgery and life for me would change one way or the other.

A week or two later, the results of the five days stay came through the post and showed that they were positive! This meant that another test would take place and I would return to the same hospital to have this done.

An appointment was made for me to go and I would stay for just over a weekend this time.

My thoughts turned towards passing this test also. I began to think further towards my future and the possibility of improvement in my life!

It was in the August of 1996, that the next tests were scheduled for. This time only a two day stay. This testing involved memory testing. When the date arrived, I packed what I needed and was on my way to the hospital.

After arriving, I went to the reception and reported in. The receptionist gave me directions to get to the ward. Making my way, I knew that I was not going to be in the same ward as the last time.

Arriving at the ward, I went to the reporting area and I gave my name. A nurse came up to me and led me to where the bed was.

A while later, after getting my things organized, the doctor who was going to be doing the tests during this stay arrived to see me.

"Hello Peter."
"Hi Doctor."

He started telling me, the tests that I would be doing would take place tomorrow.

"That's good then; let's hope that they are positive results also," I replied.

Saturday, I woke up nice and early after a good night's sleep. Later that morning, my consultant and another person came along with a trolley and asked me to get onto it. I was about to have the tests that was needed and needed to be positive for me, 'I hoped'.

When we got there, everything was ready. The consultant started to show an object to me and said to me, "Can you tell me what this is that I am showing you?" "It is a ball," I replied.

The idea was to see how quick and responsive my replies were, telling them exactly what I was seeing or hearing.

Next, they showed me a wooden toy horse and again, I was reasonably quick to reply to what it was. The consultant said to me "Repeat after me," then he said "My name is Peter."

I was a little slow to reply to repeat "My name is Peter."

More objects were shown to me to test the brain on response time.

After the final object was shown to me, the consultant said to me "That's it, Peter, the test is over," and with that, I was taken back to the ward.

Feeling relieved and now it was just a point of waiting for the outcome of the tests that had just been done.

The rest of the day, I just stayed around the ward and watched some TV and did some reading. The sad thing was that I was not going to be given the results until my next appointment with my consultant Professor Shorvon.

On Sunday, I packed everything that I took with me to the hospital as my dad would be coming soon to take me home.

He arrived at around lunchtime. "Hello son, how did things go?" He asked. "Hi Dad, I had the tests, but am not going to get the results till my next appointment with Professor Shorvon. The appointment is going to be later in August." I replied.

Grabbing my bag, we made our way out of the ward. As I did, I went up to the nurses and said "Thank you for your help and caring while I was here." "That's no problem," they said.

The day came of the appointment with Professor Shorvon. I was wondering what he was going to tell me?

My parents were also going to be coming with me to London. "Let's hope the tests are positive, it's really the last chance saloon to avoid having my bad epilepsy seizures for life," I said to them.

"We'll just have to wait and see what Professor Shorvon has to say," mother says.

We made our way to the hospital and arrived on time. Walked to the reception desk to report in, then into the waiting area and took a seat. As the waiting area was full, it may be a bit of a wait for us.

It was very warm while sitting in the waiting room, so I got up and went to buy a cold drink of water. "That's better," I said to my parent's as I sat back down to wait for my name to be called out. I heard someone call out "Mr.

Churchill." I looked up and saw a nurse standing at the doorway of the waiting area.

The three of us got up from our seats and made our way towards the nurse, as we did, she turned and led us to another section where Professor Shorvon's room was and we were asked to take a seat outside the room. "Professor Shorvon will see you shortly," the nurse said.

Professor Shorvan's door opened and he popped his head out and said "Would you like to come in now Peter?"

We all got up and walked in, and took our seats. He shut the door and made his way behind his desk. "How have things been going for you Peter?" He asked. "Still been having a few major seizures," I replied.

"I have the results of the tests that you had in July and in August and both have shown positive outcomes, as it was seen that your seizures are being triggered off from the left side of the brain that will allow you to have an operation if you want to go for it," adding "The chances of a successful operation are 70% and just a 3% risk factor."

"Well, in a sense, with all the medications that I have been through and not really anymore new ones to try, it would be the last chance saloon for me to get it sorted and possibly improve my life, compared to the one I am currently living in."

"What do you think Mr. and Mrs. Churchill?" He asks.

"Hearing what you said on what the success rate is, it's good, but it's really down to Peter in the end," mother replied.

Sitting there and I was taking all the information in and at that very moment, I was a bit undecided. This was what I wanted, yet it was a very big decision for me to make. Truly, I felt that time would be needed to sort out my thoughts and to be completely sure of my answer before giving one. This would be a life changing procedure and I really needed to feel confident in what my answer would be.

"Can I let you know in a few weeks?" I asked. Telling him "I am going for a week's holiday soon; I can think it over while I am away."

"Of course you can," he replied.

With that, the appointment was coming to an end. "I will hear from you soon then Peter." Professor Shorvon says to me. "Yes," I said as we stood up and made our way out of his office.

"Bye," Professor Shorvon says.
"Bye," the three of us said at the same time as we left the room.

"You will be a fool not to have that," my dad says to me as we made our way out of the hospital.

However, it was now down to me completely, whether I still wanted to go ahead with the operation despite the risks being in my favour.

A week after my appointment with Professor Shorvon, I went on the week's holiday to visit relations.

During that time, visiting my relatives at the seaside, there would be plenty of time for me to think, looking at the pros and con's of having the surgery done or not.

Thinking that this virtually would be my last chance in having something done hopefully in a positive way and it may just stop the epilepsy seizures. Also, the odds were in my favour.

By the end of my visit, I had decided that I would go for the surgery and 'begin my new life' hopefully. I had been reading about positive thinking and that the more positive I could be, the greater chance of having the outcome that we all were working towards in having this operation done and being successful.

Returning home, the first thing that would be on my agenda was to contact Professor Shorvan and let him know my decision.

Now it was going to be a bit of a waiting game as to when the operation would take place. We knew it would, it was just when?

The Operation

I was looking forward to the operation, the surgery was booked for November 11th.

With my parents by my side, lending their support, I checked into the hospital.

While waiting with my parent's, who had kindly accompanied me into the ward, as we had to wait for a bed to be made ready; I had a major seizure.

I was thinking after the seizure that hopefully I would become free of these episodes after the operation.

After being taken to my bed, and I had gotten myself sorted out, my parent's left me to go back home. They wanted to give me a chance to settle in after they left. As the surgery was due to take place the next day.

Next day came, and I was looking forward to having the operation. Later that morning though, my doctor came to me while doing his rounds and gave me news that I did not want.

"Hi Mr. Churchill, the operation that you are due to have today, has now been delayed until the 14th of November. The reason is due to the lack of beds in the intensive care unit," he told me.

"I had built myself up for this, so I was not happy, but it happens and I will have to deal with it and wait till then," I replied.

During the waiting time, my mother decided to stay at a hotel near the hospital, so she could see me during the week leading up to the operation date.

The rescheduled date arrived and it was time to be taken down to the operating theatre, and I was wheeled into the operating theatre. It was now fingers crossed time for the operation to be successful.

Mother was there also waiting outside the theatre, for she was going to be able to watch the operation through the observation window. As it was time to begin the operation, mother was watching through the glass window as they administered the anaesthetic. We both were wondering what was going to be the outcome of this operation? Knowing that there is always some fear or risk taken when going under the knife, it was too late now?

The surgeons opened up the side of my head above the left ear and went in with the instruments that they were going to use. They started removing the scar tissue that they could see on the lefthand side of my brain by scraping ever so slowly and delicately.

Once the tissue was removed, they placed a metal pin to hold together what they had done during the operation. This was to help stabilize the area afterwards. The operation lasted about three hours.

Mother was feeling horrified and emotional, seeing what was being done to her son.

After stitching my head back up, they moved me from the operating theatre into the intensive care unit, where I would spend time recovering after such an ordeal.

I was taken back to the ward on Friday evening. Very determined to get back out of bed and back on my feet, but when I tried to walk to the front of my bed on the Saturday, my left leg gave way and I fell to the floor.

Apparently, this was a normal thing and expected to happen as an after effect from the operation. The nurses on the ward were expecting it to happen, but I was not! Thus, I would be spending most of the time in bed for the next day or two.

Still determined to get on my feet on the floor, I started to walk about the ward unaided on the Monday, to give my legs some exercise and get the circulation back into them.

The staff and surgeons were surprised at how quickly I had recovered from the operation and that I was up on my feet already.

But I was advised not to push things too quickly in the way that I was possibly doing. The next day, I cautiously extended my walking by going around to other parts of the hospital.

After the operation, my mother went back home. During the weekend though, my parents came to visit to make sure I was doing OK. They visited for a bit, we had tea and chatted then it was time for them to return home.

On the following Tuesday, the doctor was doing his rounds and eventually came to me. After his examination, he said; "Peter, you can go home tomorrow." With a smile on my face, I said; "Thank you doctor."

Since the operation now being five days ago, I have not had a major seizure. With fingers crossed, I hoped that this was the start of a new life for me.

The next morning, I packed my things and waited for my parents to pick me up. When they arrived, the doctor told them; "After such a delicate operation, Peter needs to be kept an eye on for a few weeks."

"OK then, we will," they both replied.

This meant that I had to live with my parents for a time. As a precaution, the time there was extended and included the Christmas holidays.

Recuperating was not that enjoyable for me. Not being able to go out with my uncle, and watch our favourite soccer team play. Nor could I attend any holiday parties or lively pub and family events, as rest was the order of the weeks to come. Healing from such a major surgery takes time and patience for a proper recovery.

My Nan had come down to my mothers from Cromer in Norfolk to look after me for part of the time, but when New Year's Eve came, I spent it alone at my parent's place.

A Trip to Warwick
(My first adventure out on my own)

During the recovery time at my parent's, I made plans to visit my friend Jen. A pen pal that I had met on a social media site. Our plans were to meet in person sometime in February 1997.

'We became friends back in 1994 and had met up at my relative's hotel in Great Yarmouth, Norfolk a couple of times'.

February arrived and I was back living on my own and very happy to be back in my apartment. I started preparing for my trip to visit Jen and excited to take this trip on my own for the very first time. This trip would take me to another part of the country. As plans were well under way, I had booked a room at a Bed and Breakfast in Warwick, England.

The morning arrived for this adventure to begin. Early that morning, I called a taxi service to take me to the bus station and there, I boarded a green line coach to London's Marylebone Station. From there, I would catch the train to Warwick.

Having a nice happy feeling inside me, and really looking forward towards the full new adventure. I had never done anything like this before the operation. Plus having three different modes of transportation evolved, first the taxi, then bus, then the train. This was also going to be my very first time on a long train journey on my own!

I would have never had the confidence to travel alone on a train before, because before the operation, I was always thinking and afraid that I might have a seizure while on board.

When finally reaching the train station, I did not have to wait long before my train was due to depart. Feeling so very excited about this trip, now that I am able to travel on my own since the operation.

The two-hour journey to Warwick was pleasantly uneventful just seeing beautiful scenery and relaxing as the train went along the tracks.

Arriving in Warwick, I flagged a taxi and headed for Jen's parent's address as she was still living at home with them. The taxi pulled up and she was waiting for me at the front door with her open arms to welcome me.

We spent time chatting about many things and watched a video. I also gave my parent's a surprise phone call as they were unaware that I was going to be doing this trip to Warwick.

"Hello," mother answers
"Hi mother, I thought that I would ring you to let you know that I am in Warwick."

"WHAT!"

"I have come to visit Jen, my pen pal friend."

With that news out and mother still wondering, I passed the phone to Jen.

"Hi there," Jen says to my mother.

Jen told her that things will be OK with Peter, reassuring her.

"That's good then," mother replied.

And with that she hands the phone back to me.
"I will speak to you during the week mother."

"OK then, be careful," she replies.

"Bye mother," and with that, I put the phone down.

A little while later, we went over to the Bed and Breakfast place, so I could book-in and put my luggage away and settle into these new surroundings.

In the evening, I met Jen's parents and had supper with them and a chat.

The following day, Jen and I took a walk into the town centre of Warwick, while there we decided to visit Warwick Castle at the same time. It had a lot of interesting artifacts to see; like old-fashioned weapons that were used in the battles centuries ago, boat huts and acres of grounds to walk around.

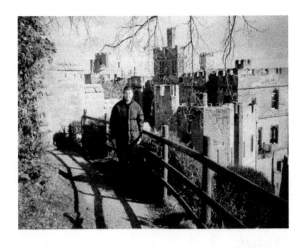

"What a nice place to visit?" I said to Jen. "Yes, it is indeed." It took us about three hours to see everything in and around the castle.

In the evening, we had dinner with Jen's parent's and talked about many things including my past and they told me about theirs.

During the week on a very wet rainy day, Jen and I accompanied her mother and went to Coventry, as she was visiting a relative in hospital.

After arriving there, during the time while Jen's mother was visiting her relative, we decided to see the sights and take a walk around Coventry's town centre.

It was interesting to see the old and the new Coventry cathedrals next to each other. While walking, we noticed it had started to rain and we were getting wet.

"We better start heading back to meet up with your mother at the car park," I said to Jen.
"Yes, we should, good idea as we are getting soaking wet."

We headed back to the car park and eventually Jen's mother arrived back from the hospital and we headed back to Warwick.

That evening, we all went to a local pub that was just around the corner from their home. It was a very enjoyable evening having a few drinks and playing pool. Jen was a good player and I told her so.

It was late when we left the pub. Arriving at their home, I said goodnight to Jen and her parent's. Thanking them for a very enjoyable time. I turned and walked back to the B&B for a good night's rest.

While lying on the bed, I thought about the events over the past few days. The life I was having felt good and I am finally doing things that I never would have attempted to do before the surgery.

The next day, we did a lot of walking. We walked everywhere, even to the racecourse. It didn't even matter that there was not any horse racing on that particular day. We also travelled to the arcades at an entertainment complex in Leamington Spa and enjoyed playing a few games of ten pin bowling.

During the weeks visit, we still had a planned surprise visit to attend to. Meeting with the ladies and gentlemen who were mostly widows that we had met during our meeting in Great Yarmouth, Norfolk in 1996.

When Friday came, I grabbed some clothes and stuff to take with me to Telford, Shropshire and Jen did the same.

With the main event of my visit with Jen yet to come, we made our way to Leamington Spa to catch a train to Birmingham New Street and then walked through a market place to get to Birmingham High Street and boarded the train to Telford.

My new self-confidence was building more and more with each new experience, having never travelled to this part of the country before.

Before the life changing procedure I had, I was having between 50 and 70 major seizures a year. Yes, my life was definitely getting better with each passing day!

Eventually, we arrived at Telford Station. From the station, we took a taxi to Woodside Estate in Telford and arrived at our friend's house. This same couple had made the arrangements for our surprise meeting with the widows. They also graciously offered their home for us to stay with them.

After dinner, we got ready, and made our way to the hall with our friends. It was in the hall that there would be live entertainment for the evening, where the surprise meeting would take place.

As we walked into the hall, the widows were absolutely taken back and also gob-smacked when they saw us both walk in together. They came up to us, saying hello and giving hugs, everyone was overjoyed to see us there.

The live entertainment started and the singer was good. We all danced and chatted the night away.

Raffle tickets were being sold and I told Jen that I would buy some for us.
"Thank you," she replied.

It was an evening we enjoyed very much. When they did the raffle draw, Jen was lucky and she won a potted plant.

Eventually, and unfortunately, it was time to leave. We said our goodbyes to our dear friends and left with our hosts.

The next morning, we had breakfast with our hosts before they gave us a lift back to the train station.

"Thank you very much for coming," our hosts said.
"It was a pleasure indeed to come and make the surprise visit," Jen replied and with that, we

headed towards the train station and caught the train back to Warwick.

Arriving back at Warwick, we parted. Jen went back to her parent's and I went to the B&B.

After a while, I spent the rest of Saturday and most of Sunday by myself. Thought it would be a good opportunity to do some shopping. I wanted to buy something to remember this trip. I bought some sweets, as having a sweet tooth also fridge magnets and tea towels with Warwick on it.

Sunday night was my last night before going back home the next morning. I spent it with Jen at her mother's, having tea and afterwards going back to the pub in the evening.

Having a wonderful evening together, it got to that time to say my goodbyes to Jen and her parent's. After thanking them for a fantastic time and all the other things, I gave Jen and her parent's a hug and said goodbye. Then I left the pub and headed back to the B&B.

Before going to bed, I packed up my stuff so that all would be ready for an early start to catch the ten o'clock train in the morning back to London.

In the morning, after having breakfast and grabbing my luggage, the owner of the bed and breakfast was kind enough to offer me a lift to the train station, to catch my train. I thanked him for it and when arriving, made my way onto the platform. The train came on time, so boarded the train and started my way back home.

On the train, I began to feel sad after having such a good time in Warwick with Jen. Yet at the same time, very happy of not having any seizures to date. It sure was a mixed bag of feelings that came over me.

Arriving back home in Hemel Hempstead around 1:15 pm. The journey took three and a quarter hours. It's certainly not a trip that I will not forget, and was hopefully the start of a completely different life to the one I'd had before.

Jen and I carried on writing to each other until about 1998, when we drifted apart, then for unknown reasons Jen had stopped writing and heard nothing more from her again.

Driving Day at Chatham Docks

Having grown in confidence since my trip to Warwick, I knew my life was improving for the better.

In 1995, I joined a local epilepsy group in Hemel Hempstead. We would meet once or twice a month to talk and socialize.   The members of this group either suffered with epilepsy or had a relative or a friend with this illness.

The group was formed to provide a greater understanding and learn more about living with epilepsy, providing them with the coping tools necessary to talk about it and to support each other.

This gave everyone the chance to express themselves and gain the confidence to be more open about epilepsy and move forward toward creating a balanced and better life.

Also gave everyone the opportunity to meet and form new friendships.

Another epilepsy group based in Gravesend in Kent, held a driving day in 1997, around the month of May. They invited other epilepsy groups from around the UK, to attend this fun day of driving a car.

The person who ran the group in Hemel Hempstead booked a minibus to take us to this special event in Chatham Docks.

We were looking forward to this outing and the chance to drive a car.

Unfortunately, one person had a seizure in the bus while we were travelling down there. Otherwise, it was a smooth drive to Chatham Docks, arriving there in plenty of time on a lovely warm summer's day.

Some of the other groups that attended this event came from Luton, Sheffield and also up north, in parts of Scotland. The event was for people who were unable to drive a car at all or were forced to stop driving due to becoming an epileptic.

The event was held on a large paved enclosed area in Chatham docks. Everyone had an instructor on the passenger side and drove a training car, (a car with steering wheel and pedals on both sides) thus being a safe place to experience what most people can do normally.

The Gravesend epilepsy group hired five cars from a local driving school for the day. We took turns to have a go at driving a car with an instructor. The area was big enough that four cars could be driven around at the same time. The experience of being behind the wheel of a car brought a great feeling of independence to everyone attending including me.

In the afternoon, the person who was in charge of the driving school gathered us all around and said that they were planning to do a competition.

The idea would be to drive in and around the orange cones that had been placed out in a line. Once through and at the other end, we had to turn the car around by backing up and then facing forward to drive through the cones again to the finish line. As this was all going to be timed and five seconds added for each cone that was knocked over, speed and accuracy was needed to win.

Since I had never ever done anything like this before, I wondered how I would do and started to get a bit nervous and excited at the same time.

The competition started and I was one of the early contestants to drive the course, with a driving instructor sitting in the passenger seat.

When it was my turn, I got into the car and drove up to the starting line. The person standing at the starting line put up his hand and shouted "Three, two, one and go," and I shot off to tackle the course.

I started weaving the car in and out of the cones until I reached the far end of the car park, with so far, no cones knocked over, so far so good. Then I put the car in reverse and backed it up how I was supposed to do, to turn the car around.

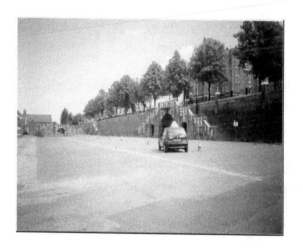

Then drove forward and started weaving my way back through the cones in and out before reaching the finish line.

Amazingly, I had a clear round with no penalties, showing a great result. I was very excited and happy at how well the performance went with no cones knocked over so no penalties added for me.

My time was one minute, eight seconds, which placed me into second place at that moment of time. But there were still a lot of people to have their turn.

Watching and waiting, seeing others drive the course, had me pacing up and down; biting my nails.

Wondering and hoping if I could stay in the top three places, that would be nice and I did have a chance. There were so many unlucky drivers knocking cones over or stalling their cars.

Everybody eventually had their turn and the end of the competition came, and it was time to hand out the trophies.

The instructor announces the results. "In third place with a time of one minute and eight seconds, is Peter Churchill."

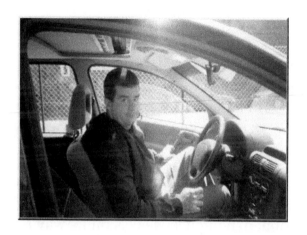

Hearing that, I was surprised and over the moon, that only one person had beat my time, and they were from different epilepsy groups who won first and second place.

The day was a great experience. It is true that epilepsy groups can help improve people's lives by socializing in different ways.

Given the chance to experience doing things that they may never have an opportunity to do.

Six months later, after that driving event, I reached a milestone, having gone one year without a seizure. I had an appointment at my local Dr's surgery. The doctor I saw, told me that everything was okay and they were happy. So, they filled in a medical form and sent it off to the D.V.L.A. (Driver & Vehicle Licensing Agency).

A few weeks later in December 1997, I received a letter from the D.V.L.A telling me that they were happy with the medical report and my provisional driving license was on its way through the post to me. Very happy indeed, another goal achieved.

I began to have driving lessons in early 1998, but after a few lessons, I unfortunately ran out of available funds to carry on with these lessons. Recalling that at the time, it was a big disappointment for me.

Finding a Job

Six months after the operation, I was ready to get back into the swing of things as in finding a job.

Across the road from where I lived was a block of apartments and in one of them lived a lady whose name was Hilda, whom I did not know personally at that time.

One day in May 1997, Hilda called my name from her balcony, as I was standing nearby and asked me to come over to her apartment. I said sure, so I made my way over to her apartment and was let in.

She introduced herself to me, saying that she was a volunteer at a charity shop called Barnardos. She asked me; "Would you be interested in working at the shop as a voluntccr?"

"Yes, I would," I replied.

"I will go and talk to the manageress then, next time I am in there."

After a bit of a chat, I decided to go back home.

"Bye Hilda."
"Bye," she replied

Hilda spoke to the Manageress and arranged an interview for me. The appointment was for the following day and my meeting was to be with Kim. The shop was in my town in Hemel Hempstead.

It was all new to me, since I had not done retail work before, and had no idea what I was getting into.

On the day of the interview, as I entered the shop, Kim was there and welcomed me in. She led the way into the small office, also doubled up as the canteen.

As Kim asked me questions, she took notes down to my replies. It appeared to me that she was thinking that I would work out OK there.

After the interview, Kim took me around the shop for a tour, explaining the things I may be doing at the shop. When we had finished the tour, she told me that I could start at the beginning of the following week.

"Thank you so much for the opportunity," as I reached out and gave her my hand. "You are most welcome Peter, welcome on board." "Thank you, Kim, I will be here at the start of next week." With a big smile on my face, I turned and left the shop.

On my way home, I was very excited to have a job, even though it was a volunteer position, it would give me the opportunity to experience what is needed to be done in a retail shop, that may in time lead to a paying job.

After having been shown the ropes and meeting the other volunteers that worked there.

My first day as a volunteer was a bit nerve racking.

Discovering that most of the volunteers were a lot older than me, and they were mostly women. They showed me how to display clothes on the walls. Also, that it was important to sort them in order on the racks by size and colour.

The first two to three weeks had passed when Kim told me that she felt I was working out very well with everything there was to learn and making good progress in the shop.

She was pleased with my progress and that I was getting along well with the other staff and volunteers. Kim then told me that she would soon start my training on the operation of the cash register. That I would be up front serving the customers and handling the cash transactions.

Being good at maths, it did not take long for me to learn the up-front job of cashing out the customers.

It would also be my responsibility to take the cash downstairs to the shop floor and place everything in order into the till before the shop opened.

In June 1997, the shop was celebrating thirteen years at its location and the local press was going to come to the shop to take photos.

When they arrived in the morning, the manageress Kim had a cake ready. She brought it down to the till. Kim asked a volunteer and myself if we would like to be in the photo with her. We both said yes, with a smile.

The three of us stood behind the cash table with the cake in front of us. The photographer took a few shots and wrote down some notes, then left the shop. The picture and story of the celebration was placed in the local newspaper the following week. Seeing this made me very happy, knowing that my family and friends would also see it.

Other jobs in the shop that were given to me included: the price tagging of the items, steaming clothes to remove the creases, making sure they would look right for sale. Also, the sorting out of bags of donations that people was kind enough to bring into the charity shop. Last but not least was to keep the shop floor clean and tidy.

To attract customers to the shop, the manageress had different themes during the year. One was a Country and Western sale and on the opening day of the sale, those working had dressed up as cowboys or cowgirls. The event turned out to be a great day for sales.

Another one of the shop's sales events was called 'Glitz'. The items that were going to be worn by the volunteers included dinner jackets, dinner suits, dresses with sparkles/glitz on them.

A fellow employee, who began working at the shop after I had, was now the Assistant Manager there. He started to look at the dresses, as he was going to wear one for the picture that was going to be taken by the local press.

For a laugh, I thought that I would do the same, even though I am certainly not a gay person. So, I looked around the shop floor and I found a glittery black dress that I could fit into along with a pair of woman's shoes.

The day arrived, and had started when the press came to cover the story. The Assistant Manager and I gotten into the dresses we chosen, and those who were upstairs came downstairs to join the others as they also had dressed up for the 'Glitz' sales event.

The photographer from the local press again started arranging us the way he wanted. We stood in a line and he took a few different shots for the news paper.

When the photographer left, I went upstairs to change back into my own clothes again!

The article and photo appeared in the local paper the following week and was seen by family members and friends. They all had a good chuckle over me dressed in a woman's evening attire and gave me a bit of banter seeing me dressed as a woman. It was all done in good fun and we had a few laughs over it all.

By this time, I had started doing my National Vocational Qualification in retail, where someone from the local college would come to the shop and watch me as I performed certain tasks.

Like putting up the displays of clothing on the walls, the displays in the front window and hanging them on the different racks in the shop.

They also watched me handling the sale and completing the task by ringing up the cash register. As the sale was completed, they also took notes on how I would reply to the customer at the end of a sales transaction.

They also asked me to tell them about the health and safety routine in the shop in case of a fire.

The lady from the college told me after doing those tasks that I had passed on Level one.

I was very happy indeed in receiving this qualification.

Once a month, the college adviser would meet with Kim, who would give her updates on my work ethics and progress.

When my birthday arrived, I had decided that I would still volunteer at the shop on that day. My lunch break came and I headed up to the tea room.

On the table, I saw a small chocolate looking cake in the shape of a soccer ball with writing on it. "Happy Birthday Peter." They all knew that I was very much into soccer and thus showed how much they cared made my day special.

I was gob-smacked when I saw the cake and over the moon filled with joy. "Happy Birthday Peter," Kim said. "Thank you, thank you all."

They started to sing Happy Birthday to me. Once again, I said; "Thank you very much."

I remember how happy I felt, just knowing that the staff and volunteers took enough interest in me and the time to plan this very special moment on my birthday.

Not everything went well for me at the shop though. There were one or two incidents.

One day, I was helping a customer at the cash register. The woman handed me a fifty-pound GBP note for items she brought that cost less than ten pounds in total. I gave her the correct change in return. However, I was unaware that the shop did not accept fifty-pound notes.

A little while later, Kim noticed the fifty pound note in the cash register and asked "who accepted it?" I told her in a nervous way that it was me who did it and explained what had happened. Kim wasn't worried; she said. "Mistakes do get made." Thank God, it was fortunate that the note was not a counterfeit and was genuine, I thought to myself. Through this mistake, I learned my lesson.

In March 1998, Kim unfortunately left her post as manageress of the shop to work somewhere else; "Moving on to better things," she said. She had been such a great manageress and a very friendly person to work with.

It was sad that Kim was going and just hoped whoever was going to replace her was as great as she was.

The new manageress was called Linda, who was a bit older than Kim was and OK to get on with. The atmosphere in the shop changed and was not the same as when Kim was there. Linda was more of a stern person.

One day, she called me into the office and asked; "Would you be interested in working at a Barnardos shop in North Finchley, London, due to the fact they were short staffed?" I replied "Yes." Since I didn't know how to get there, I was given directions on what buses to travel on, along with the bus fare to get there and back. I was looking forward to going there and gain more experience. I was starting to enjoy the travel bug, since my trip to Warwick.

The Saturday that I was going to London came, and I was up early. Nothing different for me, as I was an early riser in getting up and so got dressed and ready to go and caught my bus.

Feeling very excited for I would be having a new adventure again, working at a shop in London.

Keeping an eye out for the bus stop and looking for Brent Cross, London. When I finally saw that the next stop was Brent Cross and I then pressed the buzzer to stop the bus.

I had to make a connection to take me to North Finchley. The wait time was short and when the bus arrived, it was a red London double decker bus. How exciting to ride on the double decker bus and it arrived on time also.

I had no trouble in finding the charity shop. The Manageress Sue arrived and said "Good Morning, you must be Peter." "Yes, that's right."

She mentioned that I was going to work on the cash register for the day.

There would not be a lot of difference in each shop as all the Barnardos shops were run in the same manner.

Every so often, Sue would come from the back of the shop and ask; "Is everything OK?" I replied "Yes, thank you."

During my lunch break, I decided to take a little walk about town, getting some fresh air, and becoming familiar with the surrounding area. When it was time, I returned to the shop and carried on with my work.

The afternoon went past quickly, as working there did not seem like work for I was fully enjoying serving customers. Before long though, it was 4 pm, and the shop was closing and it was time for me to make my way home.

Sue said, "Thank you for coming up and helping out at the shop today." I replied; "I was happy for the opportunity and have enjoyed my day, thank you," with a smile I said. "Goodbye," to everyone in the shop.

Walking out the back of the shop, I made my way home.

On my way home from London, I had plenty of time to think about what a change it made working with different people and serving different customers.

As I wanted to improve my employment status to a full-time paid position. Then one day back at the shop in Hemel Hempstead, I asked Linda, if she knew anyone who could help me with putting my resume/CV together?

"Yes, I have a friend called Carol that can help you with that."

The next day, I brought my resume/CV in and when Carol came into the shop, I asked her if Linda had talked to her about helping me with a resume/CV. She replied "yes and I can help you."

Within a few days, Carol came back into the shop and handed me a copy of the resume/CV that she made for me. Looking at it and with a smile I thanked her for the work and said that it was looking impressive.

During the summer of 1998, I decided that it was time to leave the Barnardos charity shop. I had worked there for fifteen months as a volunteer doing four to five days a week. Feeling that I needed a change, plus things were just not the same anymore since Kim departed. I decided to leave in early August and take some time off as I needed a break and recharge my batteries.

'Possibility of a Paid Job'

After coming back from a holiday, I went to see Anne at the Dacorum College in Hemel

145

Hempstead to see if she could help me find a full-time job. Feeling that now that I had the NVQ certification in retail and having some qualifications under my belt.

On the 27th of August, I had an interview at a warehouse called Bonar Pack Centre in the main industrial park of Hemel Hempstead. Anne from the college came with me for this meeting.

The reason I chose to go there was because my brother Phillip, who was eight years younger than me worked there also.

We met up with the Human Resources lady and she chatted about the company and what was involved in the job. After the meeting, we left her office and were given a tour of the warehouse.

When we returned back to the office, she asked me if I would be interested in working there. After a few moments of thinking, my reply was, "I would like to have a trial period just to make sure that I was suitable for the job as the challenge would be working on machinery, that I had not worked on before." Because of my epilepsy, it would have been too dangerous before the surgery. She says; "OK then, we will do that."

It was decided then to do a two-day trial period. I started the trial period on the early shift. There were three shifts, an early, late and night shift. I would only work two of the three and never the night shift if I passed the two-day trial period.

The job involved loading materials onto the machines that the company had and packing the finished products of packed razors into boxes.

Sometimes I wondered if the possible stress of this job could cause a seizure. For now, it had been two years without any.

Over the two days. I did not mind doing the work that involved working with a team of workers on a machine, working on different parts during the day. To make it fair, we rotated the different positions of work between three to four workers.

Taking the position at the start of the machine, it was my job to load the machine by taking the razors out of the trays and loading them so they would go through the machine and be packaged. This part of the job meant that I needed to work quickly to keep up the supply for the demand.

Part of the rotation was to allow the operation of the different areas to be fair for everyone. The next stage, I was given was the packing area. It was my job to take the packaged razors and place them into a box. This was then lifted and carried onto a wooden pallet for shipment.

At the end of the two-day trial period, I decided to extend my time there and take on a fulltime position.

After a few weeks, Ann and I met with Sharon about my progress to date. She said, "If it was not for politics, I would have offered you a fulltime job." However, by law it is mandatory to do a three-month trial period before a fulltime position would be offered.

I carried on working through the trial period, and then on the 3rd of December 1998, I had an important meeting to attend. It was an update report on my progress with my shift manager.

He told me that my work had progressed through the trial period very well and as a result the company would like to offer me a permanent position contract that they would put back to the 1st of December.

It was great news of being offered the job, and start having a regular pay cheque.

Not long after my employment started, a committee was being put together with a representative from each shift, to discuss any issues that may have come up. This was of interest to me and that I would like to be a representative, and so I applied to become a member of this committee and represented my shift. I was lucky enough to be put onto the committee.

It would involve monthly meetings held by the Human Resources person Sharon and the representatives from each shift. We would discuss such topics as workplace harassment, food and drink issues with the break room.

Each member having their say and writing down what was being said, then after each meeting, we would go to our shifts and would report to our work colleagues, telling them what we could at the time. They also would tell me what they would like to have discussed to make things better for all.

Holding the position for two years, when unfortunately, during a time that I was on holiday and had missed a meeting, an individual who had gone in my place ended up keeping the position. This did not make me happy at all, as I had enjoyed being the representative.

My health started to fail a bit, due to the speed that was needed to keep up with the machines and twisting my body to pack the goods was starting to wear on the back and pained me more as time went on.

Never had thought of it at the time of starting this job, but the battering of my body that had taken place during my childhood days was beginning to catch up with me as in wear and tear on different muscles. This started to affect my lower back that was hurting badly and ended up going off sick leave due to it.

In hindsight, before starting this job, I did not think that this was going to happen in such an energetic environment. If I had, I would have looked for a different kind of job.

When returning afterwards the company had been bought by another and the name changed to Sonoco Ltd.

Due to being off sick through the back problem, the shift manager decided to give me another job sitting at a table with re-work to do. The work involved taking the razors that fell off the machines, but were still in good order and put them back into trays.

In 2005, we were given news that Sonoco Ltd was going to be moving to Poland, possibly as workers out there would be paid less. Which meant that layoffs were going to happen.

In August 2005, after working there between six to seven years, I was laid off and the company moved to Poland.

A Holiday in Tenerife

One day, near the end of my shift at Sonoco Ltd, a young lady by the name of Jo came up to me and introduced herself to me and started chatting. She told me that she knew me from my early days at school. This happened in January of 1999, and we starting dating shortly after that.

This was my first serious relationship ever and within a few months she had moved in with me.

In September 1999, we decided to make plans for a holiday at a resort called Tenerife, on one of the smaller islands off the coast of Spain.

We both were looking forward to this holiday and for me, it was going to be my very first time going abroad on a plane.

By now, it had been nearly three years since the operation and without any major seizures.

I was wondering if what I was about to embark on would be risky, because the place that we were going to was a hot and humid country, which before the operation would be a perfect situation to trigger an epileptic episode off.

On the day of going, we were packed and ready to go and feeling excited indeed. We could not wait and had asked someone to give us a lift from Hemel Hempstead to Luton Airport.

We arrived at the airport, early in the afternoon, and headed into the airport after thanking the person for the lift.

Standing in a queue with many passengers and waiting our turn to hand over our baggage. When the baggage was handed in, next the time was to wait till it was time to board the plane.

The time was getting near for us to start making our way to the plane, but our flight was delayed due to technical problems that had been noticed and required attention before being put back into service.

After several updates informing us of the status of our flight, Jo started to get annoyed as she was so excited about the trip and wanted to board. I calmed her down by putting my arm around her and we sat together. Having to wait a long while in the departure lounge and not knowing what was going to happen or when.

Finally, at 6:45 pm, the announcer told the Tenerife passengers that they had not been able to find a plane to replace the one with the mechanical failure, and had not been able to fix it yet. And that we were going to have to stay at a hotel near the airport overnight.

Hearing that, passengers including us, were not happy at all to have to lose a day holiday. We collected our baggage and went to the entrance of the airport where we would be driven to a hotel in the Luton town centre.

In the early hours of the next morning, we were driven back to the airport to catch our flight at 7.30 am. Needless to say we were all annoyed and irritated about the situation.

My thoughts were 'At least the problem with the plane had been spotted beforehand and not while we were up in the air'. This was really a good thing in my mind and perhaps not in others.

There was a bit of a delay and we were sent to wait in the departure lounge. Eventually we were asked to finally board the plane.

When on board, Jo asked if I would like to have the window seat. "Yes, thank you." The plane departed at 10 am. with a loud cheer from the passengers. Just a wee nineteen hours delay in total. Oh well, it is better to have a safe trip.

Sitting by the window was worth it to me, seeing the 'take off'. This for me was the first time inside a plane. As the plane went along the runway picking up speed, when the plane left the ground, I could hear the wheels folding up into the carriage of the plane. To see the ground below getting smaller the higher the plane climbed. What a feeling I had!

The view was breathtaking, my ears began to hurt a bit. I was told to pop them by holding my nose and pretending to blow the nose. Nice relief to get it done. Jo was relaxed now and feeling happy, that made me feel good also. We were on our way, high in the sky and enjoying the new adventure.

The eventful flight took around three hours and forty minutes, and I was already enjoying my holiday, with no worries of having a seizure.

Arriving at the airport and landing safely, was another good feeling. When getting off the plane, we were met with much warmer conditions than England, and walked into the waiting area of the airport.

We were met by a representative from Monarch Airlines. After collecting our luggage, we were taken by coach to the resort hotel.

The hotel was located in Playa De Las Americas, and was called Las Dalius. The room was ready and waiting for us, with key in hand, we took the elevator up with our luggage. The room had plenty of space with a balcony overlooking the swimming pool. "This is a lovely room and balcony view," I said to Jo. "It certainly is," Jo replied and we started to unpack the suitcases.

We purchased an All-Inclusive package for this hotel. It was nice not having to constantly pay for food or drinks and just order whatever or whenever you wanted something.

As we were feeling peckish, we made our way to the restaurant and each had a starter, then a main meal and also a desert.

The evening was filled with a warm tropical breeze and seaside sounds. Having finished the beautiful meal, we decided to sit by the swimming pool and relax and enjoy the surroundings.

The entertainer that evening was both a singer and a comedian and the performance started around 7 pm. He started by singing a few songs to the pleasure of the audience, applauding after each one. Then he went into his comedy act.

He had the audience laughing as the evening continued.

Next, he asked for five male volunteers from the audience to take part in Mr. Las Dalius. "Should I?" I said to Jo. She replied "Yes, go on Peter," and reluctantly, I put my hand up.

The comedian spotted my hand raised and called me out, but I was unaware of what I was going to be in for when volunteering to be picked.

"This is going to be a competition of four rounds," he said. Round one had us sitting in a chair near each other with an empty chair placed in front of us. The entertainer said that "I will play a tune and if you recognize the tune, the first person to race to the empty seat and sit in it will have the chance to say the title. If correct you would score a point."

He played the first tune and I did not recognize it, but one of the others did, so they ran to the chair and gave the right answer and the audience applauded. When he played the second tune, I recognized it and at the same time another male did too, so we both charged towards the empty chair and I just beat him to it as he fell onto the floor.

My answer was right and was given a point. The audience applauded as I made my way back to my seat. Through the rest of that round, I did not do that well as that was the only one that I recognized.

Round two, and this time taking it in turns, we were given a skipping rope and we had a minute to skip as many times as we could. There were two very good skippers in that round and skipping at ease with no problem at all getting a round of applause. I was one of those who struggled having not skipped with a rope for years. The rope was catching between my legs instead of my legs jumping over it.

Jo and others were laughing their heads off watching me skip and in the end, I did just eighteen skips, it was good fun, however I came last.

Round three, and we had to do a demonstration in body building. First taking our shirts off, then five different body building moves followed by doing a Tarzan cry at the end.

I did fairly well in that round, as some of the men had skinny bodies and some were on the large side including myself.

The fourth and final round next and each one would take a turn, having 45 seconds to run into and around the audience and 'kiss' as many females as possible. My turn came and I was ready and the comedian said "three, two, one and GO." I raced towards the tables searching for women to kiss. The audience was cheering me on as I weaved through the tables. Lips ready and give a kiss and move on to another. When my time was up, I had managed to kiss 21 ladies.

One of the others knew his tactics and when he was given the go, he darted his way around the audience faster than I did, kissing the ladies, going to the tables that had mostly woman at them, thus kissing more at one time and as a result he kissed 27 ladies. The other two managed to kiss 25 and 26 females, so the one kissing 27 won the round.

Four rounds of fun and games and I finished in fourth place. It was fun and entertaining, plus enjoyable for the audience and me. Returning back to the table, Jo said "She had never laughed so much in all her life before."

After the show had finished, we relaxed on a couple of sun beds around the pool, while others swam and had fun splashing about.

On Sunday after breakfast, we decided to walk into town. Along the way, we walked along the sandy shore line. The beach was virtually empty. It was as if we were the only two people on it. What a great feeling to stroll along the water's edge and seeing the ocean waves kiss the sand.

We saw a man taken up in the air by a speedboat and he had a parachute on, that was already open, due to the speed of the boat filling the chute. In time he was lifted up, higher and higher into the air.

Leaning over to Jo, I said "Not sure if I would do that." It was our intention to have a relaxing day with much less hassle than the previous one. After the lovely stroll on the beach, we headed to town and walked around Playa De Las Americas.

Spent the morning walking and taking photos of the surrounding areas. As the sun was rising higher, it was getting warmer and we decided to head back to the hotel. We picked up a few cold drinks at the bar and headed for the pool to lounge around on the sun beds.

I decided to get my trunks on and go for a swim, while Jo stayed on the sun bed reading a magazine. I jumped in and started swimming a few lengths. I had always enjoyed swimming and this was the best ever.

The next day, we came across a mini golf park, with smiles we looked at each other and decided to have a game. Also, we took a tourist train ride, enjoying the city sites and a bit of the outer limits. In the evening, we went to a karaoke bar as we both loved to sing and enjoyed doing so.

Midweek, I was thinking that this holiday was more than I would have ever imagined. All the things we had done, the walks, swimming, sunning, singing and all the drinks and food that we wanted at our leisure. We were enjoying it fully.

One of our adventures was to go to a quiet fishing village. Upon arriving at the docks, a cruise trip was being offered. "Let's go on that," Jo said to me. Getting there just in time to purchase two tickets and off we went for a great adventure on the sea.

The first place that the boat stopped if lucky, we would see dolphins popping up from under the water and presenting themselves for a photo shoot. We were lucky enough to see them, but unfortunately had not brought the camera with us.

Next stop, tourists could take a swim or do some snorkeling. They were able to see the many colourful fish. During that stop, the staff set out a buffet, a wonderful spread was enjoyed.

Arriving back at the dock, it was three o'clock, which meant that we had been out at sea for five hours. Making it a long day by the time we returned back to the hotel.

Half way through the holiday, we thought it may be time to shop for souvenirs and gifts to take back home.

The rest of our holiday was spent in various ways as we enjoyed all that was offered to a young couple in love.

Seeing a cabaret act and enjoying the evening having drinks with great entertainment.

The heat had not affected me at all, compared to what would regularly happen if I had overheated.

Our last day and night were upon us. We decided to eat out and go for a Chinese meal, and enjoy each others company. After the meal, we walked around town for the last time.

Though we had lost a day due to the delays at Luton Airport, it had been a great six days holiday abroad. It was a nice flight home too and arrived back home safely.

Up Up and Away

Nine years had passed since the operation to relieve me of my major seizures, and I was going for another new adventure in my life!

In 2009, for the very first time, I was going up in a Hot Air Balloon. It was a special present from my family in 2008 for my 40th birthday. The family had saved up the money for me to do this.

It was a lovely day in Knebworth Park, located in Hertfordshire, where my dad and I went. At long last I was finally going to have my Hot Air Balloon ride. It had been cancelled on three different occasions, due to weather conditions. The colour of the balloon was red. I was so excited and could not wait to get into the basket.

The balloon was being filled up by the person who was going to navigate the Hot Air Balloon ride. Some of those travelling on the ride also gave a hand. It was finally filled with gas and ready for everyone to get into the basket.

Once we were all in, it was time for the lift off. We went higher and higher into the air.

The giant red balloon left the ground and up into the air we went. I was not going to miss taking pictures on this occasion, as I did with the dolphins in Tenerife. This time I made sure that my camera was with me.

I began taking pictures. It was interesting to find that I was not scared of heights at all.

It was thrilling to be up in the sky seeing the earth from such a height. We were quite a high distance up from the ground, now going over green fields, farmer fields, villages and the scenery. This was an amazing and fantastic experience!

As the trip progressed the balloon driver was explaining what he was doing, telling us about the gas that was being used, then he tried to scare us. Letting some air out, we headed towards the ground, making it look like we were going to crash. But just about two metres from the ground he pulled the lever and filling the balloon, we went back up to higher altitude. He then turned back around, heading towards where we had taken off from.

Approaching where we had started from, looking below, I could see small figures on the ground. We came down and landed with a bump.

The basket gently tilted over on its side and we all climbed out. It was a great gift and experience that I would never forget and would do it again, anytime.

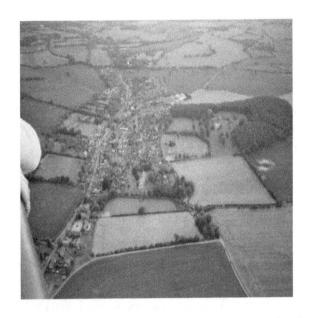

This aerial view was taken from the hot air balloon, heading towards the village. For me it was amazing to see the land below as a tapestry quilt.

Change of Lifestyle

During 2014, I became friends with a lady on a Social Media website. Her name was Telsie and she lived in Canada.

We would chat every so often on the internet, as she is a person who liked helping others.

Having her own website called 'The Orb'. There, she wrote about alternative healing, and building a strong spiritual connection for guidance, also documenting hers and others personal healing journey.

As time went on, we drew closer to each other and become really good friends.

Things started to become closer in October 2015, when we really began to become more than just friends, despite being an ocean apart from each other.

Telsie asked me once during a phone call, if I had heard of Skype and would I be interested in setting it up to chat live to her. I had never Skype with anyone at that point. A day or two later, we began to Skype each other from that point onwards, seeing each other face to face. When you Skype someone, it's virtually the same as if the person you are talking to is actually sitting at the other side of the same table as you.

Anyway, this was my first experience doing this and it was better than just texting or emailing someone. We could see the reaction on our faces and the eyes told a story that our connection was becoming stronger and stronger.

As time went on, we drew closer despite the fact that we lived in two different countries, England and Canada. 'Could there really be anything in this as in a loving relationship?' I wondered.

Telsie could see that I was a kind, caring and polite person and I could see that she had the same qualities too.

To find out if our feelings were real, we agreed to spend a month together to see if we could live under the same roof. That it would be a good idea to meet in person and arrangements were made for me to travel to Canada. Flying out on the 29th of December 2015. The visit was for a month and I would stay at her home.

Christmas is an important holiday for my family, so I would be there with them, perhaps for the last time if things worked out.

With what was to come, doing my first ever flight, whether it was going to cause any issues with the epilepsy despite not having any major fits now since the operation in 1996.

When I told my family about the upcoming trip, they did get a bit worried about me going to Canada. It was so far away and that I had lived no further than a twenty-minutes walk away from my parent's since leaving home in 1991.

I had arranged for a taxi to take me to Heathrow Airport very early on the 29th

December to catch my flight. Arriving at Heathrow Airport and moving through the line, luggage handed in and security check done, there would be a three hour wait till boarding the plane.

Those three hours soon went by and once boarded, I found my seat and happy to have a window seat. Before takeoff, I made one last text message to Telsie, letting her know that I was just taking off from the UK and that the flight was going to take around six to seven hours.

The engines started to rev up and the plane was speeding along the runway until getting up to the speed that was needed and the wheels of the plane left the ground. Higher and higher into the sky, seeing the buildings get smaller and smaller below. What an experience once again to have. This was to be my first time travelling alone in a plane ever.

Meanwhile, back in Canada, Telsie was starting to get excited about meeting me for the first time. During the flight, I put my watch back by four hours to the time it was in eastern Canada.

Knowing the distance, Telsie had to drive from her home to the airport, I knew approximately when she would set out to drive there and bring her to the airport and our first face to face meeting.

With the knowing she was driving to meet me and I was flying to reach her, I was getting excited and looking forward to our meeting.

Telsie drove for an hour and forty-five minutes before reaching Halifax Airport, where I was going to land. The flight was almost over and the plane started to descend down from the sky.

There was snow lying on the ground as a snow storm was going on. The pilot of the plane went down towards the airport as the passengers held their breath, then gave a cheer when the wheels touched down onto the runway and the plane landed safely.

Once the plane pulled into the assigned place, it took a few minutes to prep the ramp. Grabbed my hand luggage and proceeded to disembark.

Collected my luggage and made my way through security and immigration. During this time, I knew that Telsie would be getting excited, just as I was.

Walking through the last set of doors, I saw her standing there. She was not facing me so I went up to her and tapped her on the shoulder. She turned and our eyes met for the first time in real life.

Tears filled our eyes as our arms flew around each other. Telsie said; "Oh finally we meet in the flesh."

"Yes," I replied and I placed my lips onto hers in a warm greeting.

I grabbed my stuff and we made our way to a nearby hotel as the weather conditions were too bad to drive home in.

"Welcome to Canada," Telsie said, as she waved her arm across the snowy landscape. Meaning about all the snow laying on the ground plus how cold it was there as it was winter.

When we reached the hotel, we were both hungry and decided to go down for dinner. We had ordered a bottle of wine to celebrate and when the meal was done, the bottle was half full. She asked the waitress if we could take the wine and glasses back to our room. The waitress replied, "Why of course you can. Enjoy."

Next morning, after breakfast we left the hotel and made our way to Telsie's home. Now the overwhelming feeling of a new adventure was certainly creeping in and the adventure had begun from the beginning of yesterday morning in the UK.

On route to Telsie's place, she said "That it was well away from the nearest town and was out in the countryside, where many spring fed lakes could be seen." Up until now, I had just lived in a town all my life and never experienced country living on a quiet spring fed lake before and forest/woodland all around.

When we arrived at Telsie's home, we took the luggage from her car and into her home.

"Welcome to what could be your new home," she said.

"Thank you," I said.

As time went on, we were getting along very well with each other and with loads of snow laying about and falling almost every day.

I helped her with the shovelling of the snow from the walkways and front and back decks.

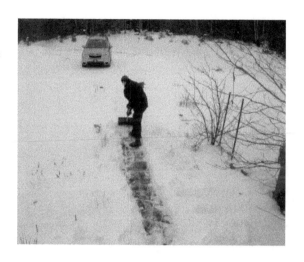

This was my first experience of living in Canada during the winter months.

Telsie wanted me to meet her neighbours and very good friends. She arranged for a dinner evening for them to meet me and have an enjoyable time.

Our trial period had started. Telsie had already thought that this relationship was going well enough for us to live with each other as a couple. As she could also see that we were matched as in the many things we had in common. But could I avoid getting anything like homesickness from being so far away from my family?

On December 31st 2015, we rang in the New Year 2016 and what a year 2016 was possibly shaping up to become.

One afternoon along with Telsie's friends, we went to the movies to see a film called "Amy." They had season tickets and I was lucky that one showing fell on the time of my visit.

We also did things like couples do, going shopping and out for a meal. Helping out when needed and spending time to chat and get to know more about each other.

Telsie's neighbour told her that they had tickets for a sledge hockey event and would we like to go. This was a fantastic opportunity to attend this special event, being held in the town closest to her place.

This was a tournament between four countries and the tickets we had would be to see the game between the USA and Canada.

If you have never heard of or seen Sledge hockey, I will attempt to explain it.

Sledge hockey is for amputees and is played with a special seat skate. It is like a sled that amputees would sit on and be strapped to the sled type skate. They use two short hockey sticks regular at the bottom and at the top end there is a pick. They flipped quickly between the two ends, when the pick end is down toward the ice surface, they thrust themselves forward and push back, thus propelling them forward with great speed. Along the way as they reach the puck with great flair that you can't even see them flip the stick around, they would shoot the puck forward to another player or towards the goal.

As the saying goes in regular hockcy, hc shoots – he scores and the crowd cheers.

This was my very first time in seeing any type of hockey game. I knew about the regular hockey and how popular it was in North America.

Sledge hockey was very exciting and we found it great entertainment. The players were fantastic at the game and the crowds very enthusiastically cheering them on.

We were expecting a great game. It was not as physical as regular Ice Hockey, yet still fast enough, with many goals attempts shot at both ends of the rink by both teams.

Definitely, we were not disappointed as the game went the full distance including overtime and penalties. Canada came out on top 3-2.

The crowd went wild of the home team winning, waving banners, cheering as we did too.

Thinking if the opportunity came to us again, we would go to another game and support the teams.

~~~~~

About three weeks into my visit now, we had a discussion on our feelings and find out if it would be possible to get married before my return flight back to the UK on the 2nd of February 2016. That would be a big step for me, having never been married before.

Following the discussion, it was decided that we were compatible enough and that we could live with each other under the same roof.

I asked Telsie, "Will you marry me?" "Without a doubt," she replied; "Yes I will," along with a wink and a smile. We sealed it with hugs and kisses.

We called my parent's a few days later to break the news to them. Needless to say, they being surprised would be the understatement.

Knowing that my mother would be worried about this trip and now with this news of marriage would be a shocker.

She had worried about me all my life, more so than the other children due to my epilepsy. Yet it is my life now, and I have had enough hurdles to climb over that got in my way throughout my life. It was my strength and belief that allowed me to move forward and make this big change to move to another country and marry the woman I loved.

We decided to get married on the 29th of January 2016. It was going to be held at Telsie's home. Invites were starting to be sent out to Telsie's neighbours and friends and a Justice of the Peace was contacted to do the service.

There were papers to be filled out and signed and a marriage licence to arrive in time.

As the wedding date came closer, I was getting nervous having not been down this road before of getting married and the possibility of going to live abroad.

The day of the wedding came and the weather was not going to cooperate, as a storm front moved in and snow started falling the night before. I had shovelled out the steps and walkway several times. Telsie was busy preparing food for the wedding guests and making sure all was in order.

She also worried as more calls came in from invited guests to say that they would not be attending, due to the bad storm. This grew to the point where she thought that maybe the Justice of the Peace would not make it either.

Shortly after saying that to me, that call came in and she spoke to the Justice of the Peace and was informed that they would be here for sure. That they had a big four-wheel truck with four-wheel drive and they would have no problems making it to our home.

In late afternoon, after my final shovelling, I started to get ready for mine and my first ever to be wife Telsie's special occasion.

Early evening and the snow had not stopped all day and the neighbours arrived by walking through the snow. They were the only guests that came because they could walk over and not have to drive.

Then a little later, the Justice of the Peace arrived, on what certainly was going to be a white wedding, outside anyway.

My family was not going to miss out despite being in the UK and four hours ahead making it 11:30p.m their time as the wedding was going to start at 7.30pm Eastern Canadian time.

They were going to witness the ceremony by phone, that would be placed between where the Justice of the Peace and we were going to be standing. The phone would be on the speaker for them to listen. The cell phone was also placed on the table for Telsie's sister to listen to the ceremony.

The family in the UK had a bottle of wine ready to give a cheer and toast to our marriage.

Also, Telsie's sister had some bubbly for a toast. It was lovely to have those from afar with us on this very special occasion.

With a total of fifteen people at the wedding, seven by long distance phone and eight at our home, thus I began my final minutes being a single man.

The Wedding Ceremony
January 29, 2016

This couple have come here today to be joined in marriage. The essence of this commitment is the taking of another person in his or her entirety as lover, companion and friend.

It is therefore not a decision to be entered into lightly but rather with great consideration and respect for both the other person and oneself.

Love is one of the highest experiences we human beings can have and it can add depth of meaning to our lives. The day-to-day companionship, the pleasure in doing things together or in doing separate things but exchanging experiences, is a continuous and central part of what a married couple who love each other can share.

Marriage symbolizes the intimate sharing of two lives, yet this sharing must not diminish but enhance the individuality of each partner.

Peter and Telsie, your marriage is intended to join you in a relationship so intimate and personal it will change your whole being. It offers you the hope and indeed the promise of love that is true and mature. To attain such love, you will have to commit yourselves to each other freely and gladly for the sake of a richer and deeper life together.

Peter and Telsie, do you both solemnly declare that there is no lawful impediment to you marrying one another here today? If so please say 'We do'

Peter, please repeat after me:

I call upon all persons present
To witness that I Peter Churchill
Do take thee Telsie Boese
To be my lawfully wedded wife

Telsie, please repeat after me:

I call upon all persons present
To witness that I Telsie Boese
Do take thee Peter Churchill
To be my lawfully wedded husband

May I have the rings that Peter and Telsie have for one another?
(Somebody places them loose into my hand)

These rings are the symbol of the bond that has formed through your relationship and is sealed in your exchanging of vows here today. Just as the ring has no beginning and no end, so is the commitment you have made to one another.

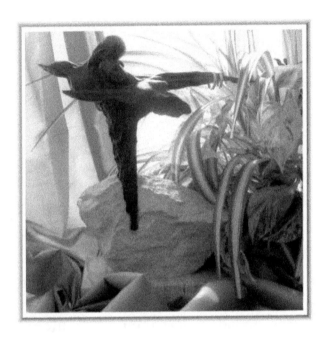

Peter, please take the ring you have for Telsie and place it on her left ring finger and repeat after me:

With this ring
I thee wed
I shall love honour and cherish thee
And this ring shall be the symbol of my love

Telsie, please take the ring you have for Peter and place it on his left ring finger and repeat after me:

With this ring
I thee wed
I shall love honour and cherish thee
And this ring shall be the symbol of my love

By virtue of the authority vested in me by the Solemnization of Marriage Act, I hereby pronounce you Peter and Telsie to be husband and wife.

May you enjoy length of days, fulfilment of hopes and dreams as you day by day live to fulfil the terms of this covenant you have made with one another. Peter and Telsie you may kiss one another to seal this marriage!

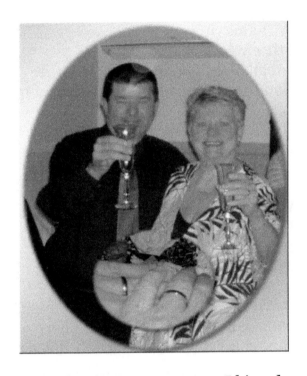

After the rings were put on, I kissed my bride, now my new wife Telsie.

There was a cheer from those witnessing this loving event in our home and those at the other end of the phones who were back in the UK and Ontario, Canada.

We both picked up the phones and talked to our family members. While those in attendance also cheered.

Someone went into the kitchen and popped the bubbly, filling the glasses. We both said our goodbyes to the families on the phone.

We were handed our glass of 'Bubbly' and were toasted by the friends that had gathered. Cheers my love, Cheers to you. Cheers to all.

Food and wedding cake placed on the table then the celebrations began.

Feeling sorry for those that could not come due to the weather, however happy for those that did and the wedding would go ahead as planned. We enjoyed the rest of the night until it was time for our neighbours and the Justice of the Peace to go home.

The next morning, I woke up first on what was going to be my first full day as a married man. Telsie woke up not long afterwards.

"Good morning, Mrs. Churchill," I said, "Good morning darling," Telsie replied.

Whoever thought that this day in my life was going to come along with what has gone on throughout it, with the epilepsy dominating it? How could I think that anything this wonderful in my life would be possible? I had always envisioned a happy ending to many of my dreams and they really did come true.

With no chance of going out anywhere due to the snowy conditions outside, our first day being married was spent shovelling the snow 'AGAIN' on the deck and the footpath. "Happy Honeymoon Dearest," my wife said with a smile and a wink.

Telsie planned wonderful meals for us to enjoy, as she is a great cook. I have yet to be disappointed at any meal.

I started to pack what would be needed to take back with me to England to settle up my apartment and clear it out. I left a lot of my things in our home, as I would return as soon as possible for Canada was going to be my new country and home.

Telsie was not looking forward to my leaving, as she loved me that much. She was going to miss me during my absence. I felt the same way but this had to be done.

Tuesday 2nd of February 2016 came along and Telsie took me back to the airport to catch my flight. It was going to be a night flight and I would arrive in the UK the next morning.

Arriving at the airport, we got as far as where Telsie could go with me, then we gave one last hug and kiss to each other saying goodbye.

I made my way to the departure lounge and eventually, the time came to board my flight back.

Arriving safely back, I had ordered a taxi to pick me up and take me back home to my apartment.

During the days of cleaning and sorting things out, I was packing up boxes and sending things through the post to my new address in Canada. Also, a helping hand from family members to get my apartment emptied.

Telsie was missing me as a result of my stay there and wanted to have me back, ASAP.

I ended up staying in England for around three weeks getting things done.

Just before I was going to fly back to Canada, the family planned a good bye gathering for me, including aunties and uncles that took place at my brother's new home, as he had just moved at the same time. Everyone wished me the best of luck in my new married life.

On Tuesday 23rd February, I took my flight back to Canada.

Telsie was waiting at Halifax Airport, Nova Scotia as I flew in from Heathrow in better weather conditions than before.

Moving through security and immigrations was the same as before and soon I passed through the doors, seeing my wife waiting and looking happy to see me. She grabbed my hand and pulled me into her for a big kiss.

"Let's go home dear and properly start our married life," Telsie says. We would live together in a quiet area that had peace and tranquillity with a spring fed lake.

"Welcome to Canada and welcome home my dear," she says, as she reached the front door of now our home. "Thank you, Love," I replied with a hug.

A Second Driving Attempt.

It was now 2020, and having lived in Canada now for nearly five years, I and my wife Telsie had decided that it was time that I thought about getting a driver's licence.

Living about twenty kilometres/miles away from the nearest town and no buses or train services where we were living.

So, in September 2020, I went to the place in the nearest town Bridgewater, where you would go and book for a written driver's test.

As it would have been since 1998, that I last had driving lessons, but ran out of money after a few lessons to continue on with them and so decided to use public transport where I was living in the UK at that time.

But now was a different cattle of fish saying wise, as you do really need to be able to drive when living in areas like I and Telsie was.

Before I was going to attend the written test, I spent time at home studying a book with everything that you need to know relating to driving from a learner driver to an experienced one.

Eventually, the day had come to go and take the written test, so my wife Telsie drove me there on the fourth of October.

First thing that was done was having my eyes tested and had to look into a kind of binocular things and was asked if I could see certain things that were shown to me and I replied yes.

I fortunately passed this and was able to move on to doing the questions.

I was handed some sheets of paper that had questions on them for me to take as it was not going to be done on a computer.

Questions were relating to signals on the road, road signs, when needing to stop, such as approaching a school bus that is dropping a child off or picking one up and having to stop so far apart from the bus. Also knowing the punishment that you could get when involved in an incident on the road while driving. Plus, other things too.

I had a certain time limit to answer the questions on the sheets, and answered them inside the time that I had. So, after filling in the sheets, I took them back to the desk where I got them from. Then went to sit down and wait till I was called.

A little while later, I was called back up to the desk and told that I had passed the written test.

Thank God for that as I did get nervous while waiting for the results.

Telsie was happy too after I told her that I had passed.

A few days later after the written test, I got my learners licence through the post and I was now able to drive our car, but only with my wife Telsie or someone else in the passenger seat as I could not drive alone.

We took it in turns to drive to places such as town to do shopping and attend an appointment somewhere.

Around early December time in 2020, I started looking around for Driving Instructors that I could look at, to start having driving lessons with and aim towards being able to drive our car alone.

So, I approached a company called 'Complete Driving School', and the person I spoke to had the first name of Debra.

We spoke and Debra asked "Could you come round for a lesson tomorrow afternoon?"
"Yes, I can," I replied.

What I was having to pay was for ten lessons plus Driving Theory Days. Twenty-five hours of classroom working (four days of six hours plus an additional hour) work also as the classroom work has to be done.

So, the following day, Telsie drove me to where the driving lessons were going to start in Bridgewater and each lesson would last an hour.

Debra introduced herself, and then pointed to the car that we were going to have the lesson in.

We got inside with me in the driver's seat, and Debra in the passenger seat that also had two pedals in the floor of the brake and accelerator pedals for her to use when need be.

So, after starting the car up, as the car was an automatic one, I put it into drive and slowly moved forward and onto the road.

Debra instructed me on what directions to take and things that I should be doing while driving, such as looking out for other traffic and pedestrians who might be thinking of crossing the road.

Up till now, I had been having practice with a neighbour out in the countryside that was pretty quiet traffic wise and now I was going to be driving through and around a busy town with each lesson that I was going to have with the driving instructor that means a lot more traffic to handle.

I went round the town steadily and took instructions from Debra as they came of using the indicator and brakes and taking turnings in an industrial estate and residential areas.

The end of the lesson came and I had not done badly.

That would be my last lesson in 2020 is next one did not happen until 12th Jan 2021.

It seemed that sometimes, my brain was taking in instructions were a little slow as my operation for the epilepsy did affect the short-term memory.

The second lesson went Ok also.

In February 2021, the first driving theory day took place as each one was going to be on a Saturday and it happened at the Oakhill Fire Department. It would start around 8.55am and last till 3pm.

Most of those that attended were mostly in their teens or early twenties. We would all sit at our own table with pen and paper and given a driving book to study from, as at the end of most sections there was a task for you to do and sometimes there was homework to take home between each class.

Over the course of each theory day, a total of three or four sections of the driving book were covered and after the fourth Saturday that I completed my twenty-five hours, it was nice to have it completed which was in April 2021. I had been having lessons between the theory days.

Between April and August, I did not have any lessons due to Covid 19 and places shut down including the Driving Instructors.

I finally had a driving lesson in August and was a bit rusty with things like over the shoulder checking when approaching stops, even though I had been driving between lessons to do things like food shopping with Telsie.

I had had over half of my lessons at this point as at the point of 22nd Sept, I had three of the ten lessons left.

So, with parts of my driving still needing some work doing on them, I had my next lesson with Debra and again going around Bridgewater.

It seemed that nerves were still getting to me, which is the last thing you need at this point.

We were also starting to practice parallel parking of at the curbside of a road or in a car parking bay (parking lot).

So, Debra would get me to turn into a car parking area (parking lot) that was in an industrial estate in Bridgewater and it was for me to start to practice reversing into a parking space, as that is usually one thing included in the driving test.

So, after getting into position to reverse, putting the steering wheel in full lock before starting to reverse around into a parking space that I was asked to park into. I would then turn the steering wheel round one and a half times so the car would be driving straight again, going forward to straighten up to reverse again into the parking space if not successful the first time.

It was hard to do as it would require taking the car forward a bit before able to have the car in the centre of the parking space.

After spending a bit of time with that, it was time to get back out onto the road. So, leaving the car parking area (parking lot), we headed back into town and turned into a side road where I could practice more parallel parking.

Debra asked me to pull aside another car that had a space behind it to reverse into. Putting my indicators on to let traffic behind me know that I was reversing backwards in a space.

I had not done much practice on this, so it was not an easy task. So, as I was reversing backwards into the space, I was parking too far away from the curb. So was asked to do it again.

Once again putting the indicators on to let others be aware and I once again reversed the car in and was a bit better, but more work required on it.

We drove back to where Telsie was waiting and I got out the car and got back into my own car to drive home.

We finally got to my tenth and final lesson on Oct 12th before the driving test which was going to happen on Oct 21st and we tackled the Motorway(highway). We had to usually use it to get from home to town or the other way round.

Being shown what to do when approaching a motorway(highway) of picking speed up so that you are going at virtually maximum speed limit when driving onto it and safely with no traffic as this is what the person doing the driving test with me will want to see. Some sections you need to yield before getting on it.

It can be a bit nerve wracking at points on the motorway(highway). So, after driving a section of it, we came back off it and back into town and did some more work involving shoulder checking, looking out for traffic and people walking.

At the end of the lesson, that was my last one and now it was going to be down to what I learned in the ten lessons and take them into the Driving test. Can I pass first time?

Driving Test Day

It was now the Oct 21st 2021, and the day had come to have my driving test.

I had been looking forward to it, but also staying calm as did not want to get too wound up and get over confident.

With the appointment at 11 am, myself and my wife Telsie made our way to where the test was going to start at, at the Access Nova Scotia building, which was in the industrial estate area of Bridgewater.

We arrived in plenty of time, then at around 11 am, a lady who was going to be my driving instructor walked up to our car. She was going to be doing the test.

So Telsie was asked to go into the Access building and sit while the test took place.

I was first asked to put the left and right indicators on, then the brake lights, and then the lady walked around to the front of the car and asked me to put the headlights on. Just to make sure that they all worked before going out for the remainder of the test.

So, the instructor got into the passenger side and belted up and then said to me that during the test, she was going to instruct me as in taking left or right turns in plenty of time before arriving at the turnings. She then asked me to start the car up and reverse the car and drive out of the parking lot (car park).

And I drove out onto the main road and down towards a busy main road.

After getting onto the second main road, I was going to drive through a school zone, and as the test was happening at a time the school was open, I had to reduce my speed limit down to 30 mph/kph and stay at that speed until seeing the sign saying end of school zone.

Next came a bit of road where I was able to pick up speed of up to 80 kph/mph and I stayed between 70 and 80.

Things were going fine so far and next was going to be on the highway(motorway).

So, I dove onto the road that was going to get me onto the highway(motorway), and so I shoulder checked to see if any cars were going close to me as I was picking up speed. I think some nerves got to me as I got onto the highway(motorway), and a very slight piece of sharp driving was made to get into the lane and had some points taken off. So carried on along the highway(motorway) until I was asked to come off it and I did so and we came to a stop sign to turn left and drive back into Bridgewater.

The instructor then asked me to turn off into a side street and as we drove along it, I was asked to park the car at the side of the road. So, I did so and it looked fine to me of how close I had parked up to the curbside.

So back onto the road and out of the side street and back into the industrial estate and I continued driving steadily and did fine at stop signs all the way through the test.

We eventually arrived back at the Access Nova Scotia building and back into the parking lot (car park), I was asked to drive around the parking lot (car park) and start and stop at certain points.

Then what was going to be the final test was reversing the car into a parking space.

It is harder than people think, and so got into position before putting the steering wheel into full lock and began reversing.

I was not straight enough into the parking space and so had to straighten the front wheels and go forward a bit before once again reversing in the space and finally got the car into the space and then turned the engine off.

The instructor said that that is the test over and started to tell me what errors were made and what points were deducted and after doing that, she said that I had passed the driving test.

I felt emotionally drained after being told that but was very happy indeed.

So, I got out the car and headed towards the Access Nova Scotia building where Telsie had been sitting down waiting and I told her the fantastic news that I had passed.

Telsie was happy indeed to hear that I had passed now. And so, I straight away in the same building went to update my licence and no longer being a learner driver, and now I could drive the car on my own when need to.

The life of epilepsy that I had endured in my life, who had ever thought that I would be behind the steering wheel of a car and on the main road. Even though this was the second time of asking, as I had had driving lessons in the UK twenty-three years ago but ran out of cash to do more lessons.

What I have done since the Operation
From February 1997
My Accomplishments

Travelled around on my own

My major seizures under complete control

Gone on vacation/holiday abroad

Worked on machinery

Done things in public
(Karaoke + competitions)

Gained lots of confidence in many areas

Came out of my shy shell

Been able to use computers

Having independence living on my own

Being able to drive a car

Passing my driving test

Hot Air Balloon Ride

Trip to Canada

Met my future wife to be

Married and moved permanently to Canada

Yet to Achieve
Anything I choose

Conclusion

Overall, my life has been full of ups, downs and changes, most of it all happening in a short period of time. I am a very positive person and am not the only person to have an illness to affect one's life.

However, this delicate operation that I had was my 'last chance' to sort out the major seizures, after having them for many years of my life.

In the telling of my story, it is my intention that I may encourage anyone that would like to see changes in their life to keep thinking in a positive way. We all have dreams and set goals, by never giving in, or giving up on a dream, and to always believe in who you are.

I did!

Whatever you suffer from, whether it is depression, mental health or Epilepsy, I hope this book helps you to get through your issues and see what you can do on the other side of the 'Rainbow!'

People who read this story might have the courage to.

"MOVE FORWARD AND HAVE A GREAT LIFE"

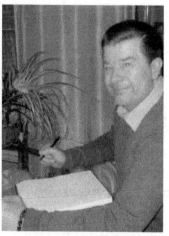

P J Churchill

Testimonial

Peter has improved his life as a result of having the operation in 1996 and has just moved forward and gained a lot of confidence to do things like travelling and even going on holidays alone.

He met his challenges head on even with the many difficulties of his condition that were told throughout this autobiography.

 Continuing to refuse to be brought down by anyone or by his condition, he aimed at targets that he has achieved and sets new goals to move towards.

In 2012, doing volunteering work for a charity called 'Hope for Children' from 2008 to 2013, each year he achieved the target of beating the amount of money he raised the year before, the charity put his name forward to be 'Volunteer of the Year' and one evening in November 2012 at a ceremony for many different types of awards handed out; Peter was announced as winner for "Volunteer of the Year."

"What a great achievement to gain congratulations Peter, well done."

www.ingramcontent.com/pod-product-compliance
Lightning Source LLC
LaVergne TN
LVHW021454220425
809260LV00001B/59